W9-DEV-066

Treatment of Chronic Lyme Disease

Treatment of
Chronic Lyme Disease

Fifty-One Case Reports and Essays in Their Regard

Burton A. Waisbren Sr., MD, FACP, FIDSA

BioMed Publishing Group
www.LymeBook.com

Treatment of Chronic Lyme Disease
Fifty-One Case Reports and Essays in Their Regard

The information, ideas, and suggestions in this book are not intended as a substitute for professional medical advice. Before following any suggestions contained in this book, you should consult your personal physician. Neither the author nor the publisher shall be liable or responsible for any loss or damage allegedly arising as a consequence of your use or application of any information or suggestions in this book.

This book may be ordered through www.LymeBook.com.

BioMed Publishing Group
P.O. Box 550531
South Lake Tahoe, CA 96155
www.LymeBook.com

Because of the dynamic nature of the Internet, any web addresses or links contained in this book may have changed since publication and may no longer be valid. The views expressed in this work are solely those of the author and do not necessarily reflect the views of the publisher, and the publisher hereby disclaims any responsibility for them.

Any people depicted in stock imagery provided by Thinkstock are models, and such images are being used for illustrative purposes only.

Certain stock imagery © Thinkstock.

ISBN: 978-0-9825138-8-0

Printed in the United States of America

Dedication

This book is dedicated to my wife of sixty-five years, whose support and love have made this possible, and to my seventeen grandchildren, many of whom are already carrying the family medical torch forward.

About Dr. Burton A. Waisbren Sr., MD, FACP*, FIDSA**

Burton A. Waisbren Sr. is a native Milwaukeean who received his B.S. and M.D. degrees from the University of Wisconsin Medical School in Madison, Wisconsin. He served his internship at the Harvard Service at Boston City Hospital. His military service was at the Navy Medical Research Institute, Bethesda, Maryland, and the Biological Warfare Center, Fort Detrick, Maryland. His residency and fellowship were served at the University of Minnesota Hospitals, where he was an instructor in the medical school. He received a master's degree in bacterial genetics from the University of Minnesota in 1951.

He moved to Milwaukee, his hometown, in 1951 and established a private practice in internal medicine, infectious disease, and immunology. At that time, he also headed the infectious disease control unit at the Milwaukee County Hospital. From 1951 to 1969, he was the director of the infectious disease division of first the Marquette Medical School and then the Medical College of Wisconsin. During that time, he was appointed associate clinical professor of medicine. He was the medical director of the St. Mary's Hospital Burn Center from 1962 to 1982. He has directed a cancer immunotherapy clinic in Milwaukee since 1973. He has published numerous articles in the peer-reviewed medical literature and has authored books on systematic methods of critical care and on medical emergencies.

---

*   Fellow of the American College of Physicians
** Fellow of the Infectious Disease Society of America

Dr. Waisbren is board-certified by the American Board of Internal Medicine and also is a fellow of the American College of Physicians and the Infectious Disease Society of America. He is a founding member of the Infectious Disease Society of America, the American Burn Association, and the Critical Care Society of America.

Recent Books by the Author

Princess Zoey and Prince Joey and Bud
      ISBN 978-1-4500-4261-1

Adventures in the Practice of Investigative Internal Medicine 1951–2006
      ISBN 978-1-4251-1328-5

The Other Princess Diana
      ISBN 978-1-4269-2504-7

The Hepatitis B Vaccination Program in the United States—Lessons for the Future
      ISBN 0-971-9351-0-6

Critical Care Manual
      ISBN-0-87488-983-9
      (two US editions, Japanese and Spanish editions)

The Family First Aid Handbook
      ISBN 0-448-14563-2

Contents

Acknowledgments

Gratefully acknowledged are the help and support of my numerous colleagues, the patients who entrusted themselves to my care, and a number of Lyme activists.

I would also like to acknowledge the dedicated help of my "attention to detail", loving daughter, Laura Stern. Without her, this book could not have been completed.

Introduction

The reader may wonder how a practicing physician from Milwaukee has chosen to present fifty-one case reports and eleven essays regarding his treatment of chronic Lyme disease.

My involvement with Lyme disease started in 1989, when the son of a woman who was dying from amyotrophic lateral sclerosis (ALS) called me and suggested that his mother's illness may have started when she developed a severe case of Lyme disease.

Intrigued by his question, I investigated by having a study done by a professor of neurology at the medical school in Madison, Wisconsin, using sera that had been collected from a number of patients who had ALS. Enough of the sera showed antibodies to Borrelia burgdorferi to suggest that a relationship between ALS and Lyme disease may be present. We reported this finding in the medical journal *The Lancet.*[1] This awakened my interest in Lyme disease, and I saw my first case in 1990.

One thing led to another, and through word of mouth and sharing my experiences on my website, I began to see patients with chronic Lyme disease and to study this disease. By 2007, I was seeing patients with this disease on a regular basis, and this has continued to occur to the present.

To my wonderment, literature began to appear, written by some of my respected colleagues, that in a sense denied that the syndrome of chronic Lyme disease occurs (see essay 4 in this book). Accordingly, I felt that the time had come to share my experience with this syndrome with my colleagues and with individuals who are unfortunate enough to have chronic Lyme disease.

This book is based on my experiences in the practice of what I had termed "investigative internal medicine" for greater than fifty-five years and my teaching of medical students infectious diseases, first at Marquette University Medical School and then at the Medical College of Wisconsin, between 1952 and 1990 [4]. Based on my initial training in infectious diseases, the medical literature, and my clinical experience, I have come to the conclusion that there is an epidemic of chronic Lyme disease occurring in the United States that warrants more attention than it is getting from the government and the academic medical establishment. It is hard for me to believe that the fifty-one cases of what I call the chronic Lyme disease syndrome represent a figment of my imagination. It will be up to the reader to make a decision in this regard.

I suggest that those who doubt that the Lyme disease syndrome exists and that it can be treated turn to the over two hundred peer-reviewed references included in summary articles written by two giants in the Lyme disease field: Dr. B. A. Fallon and Dr. Steven Phillips.[2, 3]

References:

1. B. A. Waisbren, N. Cashman, R. F. Schell, and R. Johnson, "Borrelia Burgdorferi Antibodies in Amyotrophic Lateral Sclerosis," *The Lancet* 8:2 (8554) (1987): 332–333.
2. B. A. Fallon, J. A. Niedls, "Lyme Disease, a Neuropsychiatric Disease," *American Journal of Psychiatry* 151 (1994): 1571–1580.
3. Dr. Steven Phillips, "Chronic Lyme–An Evidence-Based Review," (May 2008). http://www.ilads.org/lyme_research/chronic_lyme.html
4. B. A. Waisbren, *Adventures in the Practice of Investigative Internal Medicine, 1951–2006*, ISBN 798-1-4251-1328-5.

Observations That Surfaced in the Author's Study of Chronic Lyme Disease since 1989

1. Chronic Lyme disease does exist. It would be hard to conclude that these patients and the many others of their ilk that the author has seen are just figments of his imagination.
2. The number of unsuccessful doctor-patient relationships experienced by the patients in these case reports suggests that an epidemic of chronic Lyme disease may be occurring in this country and that it deserves more attention by the medical profession and public than it is receiving.
3. Some patients with the chronic Lyme disease syndrome may be helped by the treatment of the organisms known to be involved and by treatment of autoimmune complications, as they have been discussed in this series of essays.

Definition of Chronic Lyme Disease Syndrome

Adhering to the "Socratic" method, we will start with the definition of the chronic Lyme disease syndrome as it is used in this book. Chronic Lyme disease is an emerging infectious disease caused by at least three species of bacteria belonging to the genus Borrelia. The disease is named after the town of Lyme, Connecticut, where a number of cases were identified in 1975.

Chronic Lyme disease syndrome is suffered by some individuals who have been bitten by ticks and have not responded to the results of the bite by a twenty-four day course of oral doxycycline.

The syndrome has many aspects, and some of its sufferers have excessive fatigue, joint and muscle pains and aches, "brain fog," skin rashes, demyelinating signs, and symptoms of gastrointestinal dysfunction. Usually more than one microorganism is involved, and in some cases, autoimmunity occurs as manifested by multiple-sclerosis-like signs.

Duration of this syndrome, if untreated, may be months and even years, during which time a patient may be seriously and permanently debilitated.

PART ONE

Fifty-One Consecutive Case Reports of Patients Seen
between 2007 and 2011 by Dr. Waisbren

Patient 1
First Seen: September 12, 2007

This woman was fifty-three years old when I first saw her in 2007. She drove from Indianapolis to Milwaukee with a self-diagnosis of chronic Lyme disease associated with demyelination. She was employed as a hospital dietitian.

My examination revealed ataxia, absent abdominal reflexes, and a peripheral hyperreflexia. She brought along laboratory work that showed a low CD57 level and elevated ANA levels. She had had an MRI study that showed the white spots I have seen since in chronic Lyme disease (essay 11).

I found, with a Quest panel, Lyme IgG Western blot antibodies of 41. Quest Borrelia, Ehrlichia, Babesia, and Bartonella studies were negative. Based on her history, the physical examination, and her laboratory findings, I agreed with her diagnosis of chronic Lyme disease with demyelination and instituted a course of therapy which, over a six-week course, included ceftriaxone (4 grams intravenously), as well as Flagyl and Ketek by mouth.

This program was followed by administration of the initial oral antibiotics, changed or supplemented by intramuscular gamma globulin and hydroxychloroquine, beta interferon, and Copaxone which were selected to increase pressure against Babesia as well as to treat the autoimmune aspects of her disease (e.g., demyelination).

There was an immediate encouraging clinical response to therapy, which has continued off and on ever since. Table 1 summarizes laboratory studies that have monitored her progress, and table 2 shows all the medications that were used at one time or another.

Table 1

Summary of Lab Work

June 2003	•MRI—areas of increased signal flare in sub cortical white matter and external capsule region (essay 11)
July 2006	•Epstein Barr+ •IgM 50 •CD57 16 (ref 60-360) •Quest panel negative for Bartonella, Babesia, Ehrlichia, and Borrelia (Western blot IgG 41+) •Smooth muscle antibodies+ (1:80) •Evoked potential positive = MS
June 2007	•Western blot negative (after therapy!) •Quest panel negative
September 2007	•Liver enzymes up borderline •Smooth muscle antibodies+ (1:40)
August 2009	•CD57 low 14 •IGeneX Western blot IgM negative (41 indeterminate) •IgG positive 41+ and 39+

Table 2

Medications Given to Patient since 2006

Ketek
Amoxicillin
Doxycycline
Ceftriaxone
Rebif (interferon beta-1a)—on prior-to treatment and continued
Ceftin
Clarithromycin (Biaxin)
Flagyl
Hydroxychloroquine
Gamma globulin
Diflucan

Have we been responsible for the improvement that has occurred in the quality of life of this patient? We will never know for sure, but all concerned are satisfied with the result.

Patient History (written by patient)

In 1993, when living in Missouri, I removed a tick from my abdomen. I had a reddened area that gradually went away over a few weeks. Although cyclical flu-like symptoms followed over the next six months, I never associated it with the tick bite.

In 1996, I developed optic neuritis, confirmed on MRI which showed demyelination. In 1998, I experienced paresthesia in my lower legs, wasn't thinking clearly, and had frequent headaches. A second MRI showed new areas of demyelination, so I was given a diagnosis of MS and was started on beta-interferon injections (Avonex). A spinal tap was negative for oligoclonal bands, and blood work showed that my ANA was high.

I moved to Indianapolis in 2000. I continued to have episodes of paresthesia, muscle cramps in my legs and feet, and skin problems (rashes and livedo reticularis). My symptoms worsened in 2004 and new ones appeared. I experienced severe pain in my ankle joints at night, burning in my lower legs, very dry eyes, and drops in body temperature. An EMG showed peripheral neuropathy. I was told that my symptoms couldn't be caused by MS. My hands, legs, and feet hurt. I was extremely tired and felt utterly ill with no explanation.

In October 2005 a dermatologist asked if I had ever had a tick bite, and I remembered the bite in Missouri. He empirically started me on amoxicillin and my symptoms improved. They worsened when the antibiotics stopped. Although an initial Western blot was negative, a second one through IGeneX Lab was borderline and I had a very low CD57. I was convinced that I had Lyme disease and sought out a physician with expertise in this area and found Dr. Waisbren.

In 2007, through Dr. Waisbren, I began oral antibiotics and IV ceftriaxone for six weeks. All my symptoms went away. Three months later, they began to reoccur and oral antibiotics were restarted. This course has continued off and on. In July 2009, the joint pain in my ankles, fatigue, and generalized aching worsened. A blood test through IGeneX Lab showed a positive IgG 41 KM and a low CD57. Dr. Waisbren started me on oral antibiotics which I continued for about a year. As of September 2010, I feel well and have a very active life at home and at work.

Patient 2
First Seen: May 14, 2008

This forty-nine-year-old skilled automobile glass-replacement worker had ample exposure to ticks due to his many outdoor hobbies.

Two years before I saw him on May 14, 2008, he had suffered a tick bite on his finger. His left little finger became temporarily paralyzed. He developed ataxia, "brain fog," and extreme fatigue. His concentration was so poor that it was interfering with his meticulous job. He saw at least four doctors and underwent $20,000 worth of testing, with no diagnosis forthcoming. He turned to the Internet, which he extensively studied. He came to the conclusion that he had chronic Lyme disease. He was "*positive*" he had it. He had had several courses of oral antibiotics for various reasons, but they did not help him. His comment was, "Doctor, I am desperate and I want to be treated for Lyme disease." His complaints involved concentration, weakness, some rashes, and joint and muscle pain. On physical examination, he had some ataxia and moderate muscle and joint pains. Laboratory studies done through my office ruled out lupus and other autoimmune diseases. His Western blots, done by Quest, showed bands at 41 KD. Studies for Borrelia, Bartonella, Babesia, Ehrlichia, and other tick-related diseases were negative.

I had to make a decision as to whether to honor his phobic attitude about his Lyme disease or to not become involved with him. Perhaps unwisely, I chose the former route after explaining that the path we were embarking on was purely an empirical one. During the next two years, we tried three months of intravenous ceftriaxone, first at 6 and then at 4 grams per day. After treatment was stopped, he still was essentially disabled as far as concentration and energy were concerned. An oral program was then tried which included penicillin (3 grams per day), erythromycin (2 grams per day), Ceftin (2 grams per day), Flagyl (1 gram per day), and Ketek (400 mg twice a day). He gradually became somewhat better, so in July 2009 I suggested that he try to go back to work, which he had tried several times before. He tried and failed. He then started to talk about suicide, so his family had him hospitalized.

He received a one-week "workup" and was discharged on several psychiatric medications. On our last several visits, I shared with him that I had done all I could think of for him and that he should try "gutting" it out. I received the attached letter from him on June 10, 2009.

I will leave it to the readers' opinions regarding this case. Did he have Lyme disease at all, or had he fallen in love with the disease?

Dear Doctor,

I just want you to know how much I appreciate all you have done for me. I have been through hell on earth with Lyme disease and without your treatment I would not have made it this far. I am doing much better than before treatment, and have hope for further recovery with more time and continued antibiotics. Some days I actually feel pretty good and some not so good. I still have some very bad days, but I know there is hope. I definitely went back to work way too soon and the results were disastrous, but that's not your fault. I panicked and let the fear of losing everything get the best of me. I have to separate all that nonsense from the fact that I am feeling so much relief from most of my symptoms thanks to you and your willingness to treat this horrible disease.

I know you think I'm crazy, but I'm not. This terrible disease did cause me to say some crazy things, and I can't blame anyone for thinking I'm crazy now. If only I wouldn't have panicked and gone back to work too soon, this whole mess could have turned out a lot better. I just want to say thank-you for all you've done.

In August 2010, his sister referred another patient to me and informed me that her brother was "happy as a lark" and working full-time.

Did all we went through help him? Who knows, but at least there has been a happy ending.

In December 2010, the patient returned for follow-up. He reported that 2009 was the "best year of my life." He was energetic and asymptomatic. He felt so good that he had stopped taking the doxycycline and erythromycin that I had suggested he take for several years.

On December 1, 2010, he began to notice "brain fog" and muscle and joint pain that he had had in the several years before he was treated with intravenous ceftriaxone. He had changed insurance and had very little coverage so, at his request, I started him on an oral program that included doxycycline, erythromycin, and Diflucan. (At this time, I have stopped using Ketek because of publicity about it causing liver damage.) Within two weeks he was asymptomatic. We will continue the antibiotics for another year.

Patient 3
First Seen: September 13, 2007

This twenty-four-year-old, single, charming, ambitious young woman gave the following history: She sustained a tick bite with rash in Wisconsin at age seven. She developed severe hives after this and then generalized arthritis. A diagnosis of rheumatoid arthritis was made, but there was never any serologic evidence of this disease.

At age thirteen, she developed hair loss, chronic fatigue, and concentration issues ("brain fog"), all of which had continued until I saw her on August 10, 2008. On physical examination, she had definite ataxia and absent abdominal reflexes.

She brought in a questionnaire that she had found on the Internet which had convinced her that she had chronic Lyme disease, and that is why she sought me out.

After an examination, I shared with her my thoughts that:

1. Something indeed was wrong.
2. My differential diagnosis was between multiple sclerosis (which as the reader of these case reports will know, I had found in chronic Lyme disease) and chronic Lyme disease. (essay 11)
3. Chronic Lyme disease.

I felt that there was enough possibility that she had chronic Lyme disease that on a clinical basis, I advised that we should start treatment with oral doxycycline (100 mg twice a day), Ceftin (500 mg twice a day), and Flagyl (500 mg) once daily for six weeks. Her laboratory work showed borderline antibodies against Borrelia but no evidence of other tick-related diseases. Her lumbar puncture revealed high globulin, and antibodies against myelin were positive. This is the ninth patient in whom demyelination was suspected in this series.

When seen in six weeks, the improvement was not convincing, perhaps because of her intolerance to Ceftin, which we added at three weeks.

On August 21, 2008, she lost her job and insurance and moved to Indiana, so I sent the following letter:

To [Case 3's] Insurance Provider at a Medical Center:

This will introduce _____, date of birth November 8, 1994. I am trying to decide whether she has early MS or demyelination due to chronic Lyme disease. There was enough of a response to oral doxycycline, Ceftin, and Flagyl that I have suggested a four-week course (eight weeks if responds) to IV Rocephin (4 grams a day) along with oral erythromycin and Flagyl through a PIC line on an outpatient basis.

I have enclosed the pertinent data from her chart, and since she has moved, I suggested a "fresh start" at an academic institution.

Please send me your evaluation and plan. In my clinical evaluations, I decided that something is wrong and that we are not dealing with a "somatic disease." She and I would deeply appreciate careful consideration of this case.

Sincerely,
Burton A. Waisbren, MD, FACP

I called the patient in July 2010, and she has not been able to find a doctor who will take her seriously, although I am not sure how hard she has tried. She still has her presenting symptoms. I, of course, feel badly because in my concept of a "perfect world," she would have somehow received intravenous therapy with a possible chance of a "cure."

Summary: A case that suggested Lyme disease and multiple sclerosis.

Patient 4
First Seen: October 4, 2007

On August 10, 2007, a forty-year-old physical therapist was kind enough to summarize her case for me. It follows, although I omitted some of her feelings regarding her previous care. Her summary is in italics, and my comments in text.

I am a physical therapist. I know my body. I was healthy and fit until June 9, 2007, when I attended an outdoor party in Richmond, Illinois. A day after the party, I noticed a red, circular rash about the size of a quarter on my lower right abdomen. I knew immediately this bite was different than a typical bug bite—it was angrier-looking and had a distinctly defined center. I immediately thought of Lyme disease, but everyone I knew who lived in Richmond, Illinois, and all the medical professionals I knew said "no way." It couldn't be Lyme disease. They had never heard of it in Richmond or in Illinois for that matter. So I put it out of my mind.

About four days later, I suddenly felt very sick, faint, and out of it. I had several bouts of diarrhea. My husband rushed to my side and took me to see the obstetrician who had delivered my second baby four weeks before. He said the symptoms were probably nothing or blood poisoning. About the bite, he said he had also had one on his arm, probably from a mosquito.

The feeling of being sick remained, so a week later I saw an internist. He said I absolutely did not have Lyme disease because I hadn't seen the tick, and the tick would have ballooned up with blood to an enormous size. He also said that there was no Lyme disease in our area. He did not advise treatment or studies. Then the muscle twitches began along with the strange traveling paresthesias. Then I noted electric-type currents through my extremities and migrating joint pain.

I continued to seek help and saw two other physicians in my area. They empirically prescribed antibiotics but said that the blood tests that they had run were negative, so I could not have Lyme disease. My symptoms continued and got worse, and then a brain fog set in. I couldn't seem to concentrate. I felt mentally weighed down and fuzzy-headed and mentally depressed and frightened.

I sought another internist who, when my Lyme test came back negative, told me I couldn't have Lyme disease and that I should discontinue the antibiotics. My symptoms remained. I began wondering if it's not Lyme, then what is it? A pinched nerve, carpal tunnel, fibromyalgia, some progressive neurological disease? I was researching and researching and still, the only thing that made any sense was Lyme. Eventually, and logically, my mind wandered towards MS. By this point, I had developed a positive Lhermitte's sign. I referred myself to a chiropractor. I saw him three times, and he was stumped. But we did discuss the possible justification for an MRI. So I didn't appear to be a hypochondriac, I referred myself to a neurologist at another one of Chicago's premier hospitals prior to requesting an MRI. This neurologist, I could tell somewhat reluctantly, gave me the referral. The MRI reveals the cause of many of the symptoms—4 white lesions, 2 in the brain and 2 in the cord. He then referred me for a lumbar puncture, which came back positive for antibodies to "something" and 2 oligoclonal bands. He diagnosed me with, most likely, relapsing-remitting MS. My "Lyme tests" were again negative. My family and I were crushed. We discussed beginning MS drugs. I soon thereafter had my first full-blown neurological event, partially brought on by the stress of this nightmare—diffuse numbness and muscle spasms, and ended up in the ER, and then in the hospital for a night.

The patient continued her search for help, and more consideration of the possibility of her findings being due to Lyme disease and, through this website, decided to come to see me about her problems. Her history, the white lesions on her MRI, the picture of her tick bite that she showed me, her hyperreflexia, paresthesia, ataxia, and absent abdominal reflexes convinced me that she had Lyme disease masquerading as multiple sclerosis. An empiric course of anti-Lyme disease therapy was started through a PIC line. It consisted of a six-week course of 4 grams of intravenous ceftriaxone and 500 mg of Flagyl given twice a day by mouth. She continued on oral doxycycline and erythromycin. Blood tests done at her first visit did come back suspicious for Lyme disease. They were done by Quest Laboratories and confirmed by Bowen Laboratories. She also had antibodies against Bartonella henselae and Bartonella quintana, which confirmed exposure to ticks. Four months after the completion of the intravenous ceftriaxone, she describes her situation as follows:

I completed a six-week course of IV antibiotics, coupled with some oral medications, and am now in my fourth month of treatment for chronic Lyme disease. I feel immeasurably better. My brain fog has completely cleared. I'm not tripping over my words or losing my train of thought anymore. My paresthesias and muscle twitches are few and far between. My energy level is up. All in all, I feel almost back to normal and most definitely vindicated. And I'm now on a mission to educate others about this often misdiagnosed and mistreated disease. This is a "silent epidemic," as many like to call it. Had I listened to the highly regarded and overly confident neurologist who diagnosed me with MS, I would now be much sicker, getting precisely the wrong treatment, and headed for more debility.

Comment: Of course, a few anecdotes do not establish anything, but each case of an unusual nature that presents itself to an inquiring physician should not be ignored. This buttresses my opinion that cases of an MS-like nature which appear after tick exposure deserve an empiric course of Lyme treatment (see essay 11).

The patient was contacted on September 31, 2009. She stopped all antibiotics by mouth six months after the course of intravenous ceftriaxone (she had been put on Ceftin, Ketek, and Flagyl). She stopped because of persistent gastrointestinal symptoms. They finally subsided after she took probiotics for a month. On September 31, 2009, she felt well and was working full-time. She had some eye complaints which we will check on by an optic nerve potential test. She has no discrete neurologic symptoms.

This case buttressed my opinion that demyelination associated with Lyme disease will sometimes respond to treatment for chronic Lyme disease (see essay 7). She was followed up by e-mail in June 2011 and feels "entirely well."

Patient 5
First Seen: September 13, 2007

This was a patient who on a nature hike in December, 2006, suffered a tick bite.

Chronologic History

January 2007
   Attack of Bell's palsy that responded to one week of oral prednisone therapy.

April 2007
   She developed blurred vision, generalized paresthesia, and numbness in her lower extremities. She saw a physician who suspected multiple sclerosis. A lumbar puncture was negative for that disease. A Western blot for Lyme disease showed a positive 41 KG IgG band.

June 14, 2007
   I saw her first on this date. She had gone on outdoor camping trips for the previous ten years in tick country with no recollection of a tick bite. Physical exam showed only hyperreflexia and absent abdominal reflexes. Complaints were of paresthesia, blurring vision, fatigue, and weakness of the lower extremities. I made a clinical diagnosis of Lyme disease (Bell's palsy, paresthesia, weakness, fatigue, and absent abdominal reflexes).

Laboratory studies showed mild hypothyroidism, 41 KG IgM Western blot band, but no evidence of other tick-caused diseases or antibodies against Borrelia. I made a clinical diagnosis of Lyme disease and started her on Armour thyroid and doxycycline (100 mg by mouth three times a day).

July 23, 2007

There was some improvement in the paresthesia and fatigue, but she still felt "sick." I added Ceftin (500 mg by mouth three times a day) and Diflucan (200 mg by mouth per day).

September 19, 2007

When seen, she was essentially asymptomatic.

April 19, 2008

The improvement continued, and she elected to stop all medications.

September 10, 2009

I contacted her husband by phone, and she had just given birth to a healthy baby boy. Her pregnancy had gone well, and she had taken no antibiotics for a year. She had continued to take thyroid medications.

It seems to me that this was a classic case of Lyme disease that showed demyelinating presentation and responded to oral therapy with doxycycline (see cases 1 and 4 and essay 11).

Patient 6
First Seen: October 10, 2007

This forty-eight-year-old male had been in previously good health until July 2007. In June 2007, he had visited a deer farm in Illinois with a female companion, who developed documented Lyme disease soon after.

The history the patient gave me was as follows: A month after the visit to a deer farm, he noted his arm twitching and pain in his calf muscles. By the end of July 2007, he became "fatigued, forgetful, and irritable." On August 2, 2007, he started oral doxycycline (100 mg twice a day). He kept this up, but his symptoms did not improve, and he developed blisters on his feet. The doctor who was treating his female companion for Lyme disease started him on doxycycline, rifampicin, and Zithromax. Because he had not noted improvement, he made an appointment to see me on October 10, 2007. He brought with him a report from IGeneX Laboratory which showed a negative blood test for Borrelia and a Western blot positive for 34 and 39.

During the October 10, 2007, visit to my office, the physical exam was essentially negative for a lupus screen but was positive for the Epstein-Barr virus and CMV virus. Lyme studies by Quest showed anti-Lyme antibodies at a titer of 1.10, but negative Western blot studies (we have seen Western blot positives disappear after therapy). Studies for Bartonella were negative.

Even without the old records but with the knowledge that his female companion had been treated, I felt that a course of intravenous ceftriaxone was indicated.

The rationale for this was explained in detail, and he agreed to have a course of intravenous ceftriaxone arranged. His managed-care carrier agreed, and they chose the "Home Infusions Solutions" organization which was affiliated with Rush Medical College as the agency to give the treatment. The following program was ordered and instituted by this agency for five weeks:

1. Ceftriaxone— 4,000 mg in 100 ml of saline infused by gravity every 24 hours.
2. Lab: weekly CBC, SGPT, and SGOT blood tests; and C difficile in stool.

I saw the patient again on November 12, 2007, and he reported that the response, at best, was equivocal. We decided on continuing for another month, and this was ordered.

During the third week of this period, the patient developed a high fever and chills. He was admitted to the emergency room of Rush Medical Center, where their diagnosis of acute bacterial septicemia was confirmed by several blood cultures that revealed serratia bacteremia that responded to the antibiotic treatment suggested by sensitivity studies. As it turned out, the hospital had been notified at that time that the heparin preparation which they had been using to keep the pic line open, was contaminated with serratia bacteria. The patient responded well to the treatment for septicemia, and the follow-up suggested by the CDC was followed by blood cultures for several months, which remained negative. Of course, the PIC line through which the antibiotics had been given was removed.

The patient was understandably disturbed, and he notified me that the treatment had not helped, and that he was seeking other medical help.

I, of course, accepted this and told him that his next physician might want to treat both his high titers of viral infections as well as Bartonella, the most usual infection associated with Lyme disease that does not respond to intravenous antibiotics.

Patient 7
First Seen: October 16, 2007

This retired seventy-two-year-old army man was bit by a tick in July 2008 in northern Wisconsin. He was an outdoorsman, and his dog had been successfully treated for Lyme disease in the fall of 2007. Two months after the tick bite, which was not followed by a rash that he remembered, he developed generalized joint pain. His doctor, without an involved workup, started him on prednisone (20 mg by mouth twice a day). In spite of this, he continued to have generalized joint pain with swollen fingers and ankles. There was no clinical response to prednisone. His son, who was a pharmacist, thought he had Lyme disease and referred him to me. He had always been in excellent health and had for years indulged in, what his wife said, was a large amount of alcohol. He had never been seriously ill during many years of military service. On one physical examination, he did have tender, swollen ankles and wrists and an enlarged liver.

He was reluctant to have much laboratory work done and brought in reports that showed a negative test for rheumatoid arthritis and otherwise normal routine blood work. He was on Medicare and said he could not afford the IGeneX Lab studies that I suggested. He did consent to antibody studies for Borrelia, Western blot studies for Lyme disease, a lupus panel, and an Epstein-Barr screen, which was done by Quest. Only Epstein-Barr titers were abnormal. At this point, I can only say that in my experience this Epstein-Barr virus may be a cofactor in chronic Lyme disease.

In a conference with the patient and his wife, I explained to them that I thought there was enough of a possibility that he had Lyme disease that it would be reasonable to initiate the following plan:

1. Taper his prednisone to zero.
2. Try doxycycline, Ceftin, erythromycin, and Flagyl for a month. If there was not a clinical response, start intravenous ceftriaxone in high dosages along with empiric treatment for tick-associated diseases.

He agreed to this plan after talking it over with their son, who is a well-trained pharmacist.

The patient was seen again on December 4, 2008. The oral medications had not seemed to be of benefit. He had been able to wean himself from prednisone.

Accordingly, I outlined a plan for six weeks of intravenous ceftriaxone to be given at home by organizations we have in Milwaukee that specialize in home intravenous therapy. This organization had given intravenous ceftriaxone to several patients of mine who I thought had chronic Lyme disease. Their personnel had been impressed with the results in a few patients. I asked the patient to take the plan to his insurer, which he had in addition to his Medicare. To my pleasant surprise, the insurer accepted the plan and we were able to institute it starting in January 2009. Prior to treatment, he was essentially crippled with generalized joint pain, and he started to develop ataxia.

He then received eight weeks of the following daily: Initially a PIC line was inserted at St. Mary's Hospital in Milwaukee. Their radiology department had pioneered the PIC-line technique. Then, with me present and an EpiPen handy, he was given the initial infusion of ceftriaxone at St. Mary's Outpatient Department in the dosage of 6 grams in 50 cc of saline. I have repeatedly found that 6 grams of ceftriaxone is tolerated intravenously for long periods of time.

The home infusion team then went to his home the next day and taught his wife how to give the infusion and how to clear the line with heparin. Infusions were given during a one-hour period. The home-care nurse visited the patient weekly to check on his progress and to draw blood for a basic metabolic panel and blood count and to collect a sample for urinalysis. He had orders for a stool for clostridium difficile if he had any diarrhea. The visiting nurse was present during the first five days and then weekly. The patient's wife kept in touch with me by phone.

Oral erythromycin (2 grams daily) and Flagyl (500 mg daily) were taken as well. They were to treat empirically Bartonella and the cystic phase of Borrelia, respectively.

I saw the patient in my office on April 13, 2009. He had tolerated eight weeks of intravenous ceftriaxone at a daily dose of 6 grams without any complications given for eight weeks. He had gradually lost all joint pains and stated that he was back to "normal." He was continued on doxycycline (100 mg by mouth twice a day) and Flagyl (500 mg once daily).

I last saw him on October 12, 2009. He had no complaints. He said he had reduced his alcohol intake and that he had become his "active old self." His Lyme tests were repeated and for the first time showed a positive IgG 30 KD band. I had acquiesced to his wish to stop oral antibiotics in July 2010.

Comment: This case seems almost too good to be true, and it may be. However, we ended up with a well man who was completely disabled before therapy. The okay from his insurance carrier without a "peep" almost seems too good to be true, as well.

Patient 8
Seen: October 17, 2007

Patient 8, seen October 17, 2007, is the first case of Lyme disease that I saw in Milwaukee. This case is of particular interest because it best illustrates the course of chronic Lyme disease which was untreated over a four-year period before first I saw her in 2004. She developed a heart block six years later.

The patient is a forty-one-year-old English teacher who at age twenty-two, because she was in the National Guard Reserve, went on maneuvers at Fort McCoy, an army base in Wisconsin which is in the heart of Lyme country. While sleeping in a tent, she sustained a tick bite on her abdomen. One week later, she developed a rash on her abdomen that was associated with a low-grade fever, muscle and joint aches, and some swelling of her ankles. These complaints continued for the next four years, until she was treated for Lyme disease.

A dermatologist diagnosed the rash as ringworm, and her personal physician could not make a definitive diagnosis, so he gave her an empiric course of prednisone that started with a dose of 30 mg per day and was tapered to 10 mg per day. All symptoms continued, and after eight months, he referred her to an infectious disease specialist. She had an extensive workup, and it was concluded that she had a chronic connective tissue disease. She referred the patient to the Medical College of Wisconsin for further testing. The Lyme disease test that the infectious disease consultant performed was negative, and she discontinued the idea of Lyme disease on this basis. However, in her report she stated, "If all further tests are negative, it might be worthwhile to try an empiric treatment for Lyme disease."

During the next four years, the patient was under the care of the Specialty Services of Medical College of Wisconsin. She was seen in succession by the general medicine, rheumatic disease, hematology, and infectious disease specialty services. The rheumatologist tried a course of methotrexate which did not help.

During this time, the diagnosis of the specialty services of the medical school was that she had adult-onset Still's disease. This intrepid woman continued her education, graduated college, and started to teach English.

I first saw her in consultation in January 1994, at the suggestion of her mother. She appeared chronically ill, had a low-grade fever, and had tender and slightly swollen ankles. After a prolonged history and physical exam, the diagnosis of chronic Lyme disease seemed to me the best possibility, so I started her on doxycycline at a dosage of 100 mg twice a day. My opinion was that if the doxycycline did not alleviate all symptoms, an intravenous course of ceftriaxone would be in order. (The record of her 1993 Lyme antibody study is lost, but as I remember it, a high titer of anti-Lyme disease antibodies was found.)

The patient had improved somewhat when I saw her six weeks later, but she was by no means cured. Accordingly, it was arranged through the outpatient department of St. Mary's Hospital for her to receive 4 grams of ceftriaxone intravenous daily for four weeks. When this was discontinued, she was placed on oral doxycycline (100 mg) by mouth for the next three months.

All of her symptoms and signs gradually normalized. She regained her normal weight and resumed a daily jogging routine that was dear to her heart. Her Lyme antibody test done by Quest at that time was negative, and tests done to monitor her tolerance of the therapy were normal.

I did not initially repeat the intensive laboratory workup that had been done at the medical school. The patient has continued to be seen in follow-up since her initial visits.

In August 1994, she developed a septic arthritis of her right ankle which responded to intravenous lincomycin and gentamicin. We were unable to culture an organism from the joint, so she was given another six months of doxycycline.

She continued to lead an active life until 2007, when she developed incidents of syncope. It was found that she had a complete heart block which necessitated a pacemaker, which is still functioning well under the monitoring of her cardiologist. Hers is the second heart block I have seen develop after Lyme disease. The first was in a four-year-old child who also needed a pacemaker. Heart blockage is a known complication of Lyme disease.

Starting in 2004, her compulsive jogging started to catch up with her, and she needed reparative surgery to one of her hips. A Lyme panel done in 2010 was negative. It included Bartonella, Ehrlichia, and Babesia, Western blots for IgG and IgM, Lyme disease, and antibodies for Lyme disease. When I last did a complete exam in April 2010, she was a vibrant, well-functioning young woman with a hip problem.

Patient 9
First Seen: October 25, 2007

This very stable factory worker had worked herself up to a supervisory position by dint of hard work, good health, and dependability. Up to the late summer of 2001, her only health problem had been some difficulty with back pain, which apparently was due to some disk problems in her mid- and lower back. In August 2001, while vacationing in northern Wisconsin, she suffered three tick bites, one on her neck and the other two on her upper arm. Within a week, she had developed rashes which were described as typical bull's-eye rashes. (Figure below)

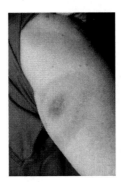

Concomitant with this were a low-grade fever, fatigue, and rather severe generalized joint pain. About a month later, she consulted her physician, who suspected Lyme disease and ordered blood work. It was done by Quest Laboratories and showed antibodies against Lyme disease at a level of 1:50 and Western blot bands positive at 21, 41, 45 KD IgG, and positive at 23, 41 KD IgM. He gave her a course of doxycycline for ten days.

In spite of this, she continued to have generalized joint pains, low-grade fever, and "brain fog."

She was acquainted with a patient of mine who had a similar experience and who, after self-diagnosing herself as having Lyme disease, had seen me and had gotten better after a four-week course of intravenous ceftriaxone. Because of this, she decided to see me. (Her acquaintance is patient 11 in this series.)

I saw this patient for the first time on January 15, 2003. On physical exam, there was moderate swelling and tenderness of her ankles and wrists. Because of my experience with her friend who had referred her, I did a careful neurologic exam and found some hyperreflexia, absent abdominal reflexes, and some unsteadiness on her feet.

During the next three months, she was given 4 grams of intravenous ceftriaxone for four weeks on two successive occasions. The response was not spectacular but somewhat encouraging. I kept her on Ceftin, doxycycline, and Flagyl in usual dosages. However, as 2003 progressed, she became more unsteady on her feet and had more hyperreflexia and more fatigue. As this progressed, a demyelinating element to her disease seemed to rear its ugly head. In addition, she was beginning to have vision problems.

An MRI of her brain revealed the following: "scattered increased intensity within the deep white matter in the right and left frontal and parietal lobes—they are nonspecific and can be seen in multiple sclerosis, Lyme disease, and in atrophy of the brain" (see essay 11).

By this time, she was becoming plagued with insurance and work problems of the type one sees often with insidious chronic diseases. She was fired and lost her insurance. She had to get an attorney to get a settlement for the way her company treated her, which helped a little. However, her care during the last nine years has necessitated the help of pharmaceutical companies and another organization that helps people in her straits and who helped in getting her through an eighteen-month stressful time in getting on Medicare because she had become disabled.

By this time, I felt that she needed empiric treatment with Copaxone for the demyelinating aspects of her disease and multiple oral antibiotics to combat the Borrelia that theoretically were active in her body— doxycycline, Biaxin, and Diflucan. After eighteen months of daily Copaxone, she had an anaphylactic reaction to the Copaxone, so we switched her to beta interferon.

During the last six years as the above medical program was being orchestrated, her situation stabilized to less fatigue, less ataxia, better vision, and somewhat less difficulty with chronic joint and muscle pain. Her most recent MRI showed probable improvement in the white spots. The oral antibiotics were gradually stopped.

The last visit on October 25, 2010, was the most satisfying visit with her I had ever had. An MRI done at that time was reported as showing an improvement in the central nervous system findings.

She has stopped antibiotics. She is still taking beta interferon once a week and takes occasional Ultram for pain. This now is all that she needs for pain. All in all, she seems well.

At this point, it seems to me that she did have chronic Lyme disease which might well have been the cause of the demyelinating disease. Hopefully, the Borrelia finally has been eradicated and the atypical demyelinating disease may be dying out. From a clinical standpoint, she and I are satisfied with the present situation and feel that what she went through might well have been worthwhile (see essay 11).

Patient 10
First Seen: November 15, 2007

This forty-one-year-old woman who held a master's degree in neurology from Northwestern University was bitten by a tick in the summer of 2001 in northern Illinois. The bite was followed by what her research showed was a typical bull's-eye rash (See figure from Patient 9).

Within two weeks, she noted that something was wrong with her. It started with localized neck pain and progressed over the next three years to "brain fog," paresthesia over her lower extremities, severe headaches, right-sided weakness, and fatigue that was so overwhelming that she could barely function enough to care for her two small children.

She saw a succession of doctors who were unable to make a diagnosis. She, using her scientific training, went to the Internet and made the diagnosis of chronic Lyme disease. One of her doctors, who thought she probably had early multiple sclerosis, did blood tests for Lyme disease which were "negative." He did not think she had Lyme disease, but she prevailed upon him to order a month's course of doxycycline (100 mg given twice per day). She noted definite improvement, but when the doxycycline was stopped, her fatigue, "brain fog," and paresthesia returned. He agreed to another two months of doxycycline at a dosage of 400 mg per day.

This time there was again a response, but when it was stopped, her neurological and concentration problems, as well as extreme fatigue, returned. She noted the acceleration of her problems to occur after she received a tetanus injection for a scratch that occurred after she worked in her garden. Her doctor did not want to go further, so she turned to "health food" medication which included a mushroom preparation. When this apparently caused liver enzyme elevation, she discontinued this and went back to the Internet, where she found my website and called for an appointment.

She was seen first on January 18, 2005. It seemed apparent to me that this was a brilliant young woman whose complaints had to be taken seriously. Her physical examination was essentially normal, although she did have some right-sided weakness and paresthesia along the right side of her body. Pain points for fibromyalgia were not present.

Laboratory studies revealed borderline-low T_3. Antibodies from Borrelia, Bartonella, Babesia, and Ehrlichia were not present (Quest). Western blot studies for Lyme disease were negative (Quest). A complete autoimmune panel by Quest revealed antibodies against smooth muscle in low titer, and titers against the Epstein-Barr vaccine were elevated. She told me that an MRI for signs of multiple sclerosis in her brain was "negative" for that disease. She did not want to get another MRI.

I saw the patient again on February 13, 2005, and I wrote out for her an initial evaluation and plan after our initial two-and-a-half-hour session, after I reviewed her laboratory studies:

1. You may have gotten to the point that you are concentrating on your body so intensively that medically insignificant things have come to the fore. I do not think that is the case.
2. You may have masked hypothyroidism because of your "brain fog," and fatigue may be due to the fact that your pituitary gland has not responded enough to your relatively low T_3 with TSH.
3. Your bizarre findings might be due to chronic Lyme disease. That is my best guess as to what is happening.
4. You may have an element of the chronic fatigue syndrome as suggested by your high antibody titer against the Epstein-Barr virus.
5. There may be an element of autoimmunity in your case which we will keep in mind (antismooth muscle antibodies).

I suggested an empiric treatment for the possibility of chronic Lyme disease and for masked hypothyroidism. This would be doxycycline

(100 mg twice a day by mouth), Ceftin (500 mg twice a day by mouth), Armour thyroid (2 grains twice a day by mouth), and Flagyl (500 mg by mouth daily) to treat the cyst phase of the Lyme spirochetes and to prevent fungus growth in the bowel.

I also wrote, "If there is no response to this, I will seriously consider with you a six-week course of intravenous ceftriaxone given on an outpatient basis. In addition, we will suggest a lumbar puncture and MRI of your brain to rule out early multiple sclerosis." We never had to go to this program.

The patient accepted the idea of the empiric treatment of chronic Lyme disease and masked hypothyroidism, and prescriptions were written and she started on the treatment. She was given the program mentioned above for the next six weeks.

We kept in touch by phone, and things seemed to be going well, both in regard to tolerance and amelioration of most of her symptoms.

I saw her in the office since then on May 24, 2005; September 29, 2005; January 11, 2006; January 12, 2006; July 08, 2006; January 7, 2006; and November 2007. We monitored her basic metabolic panels, blood count, and urinalysis, and tolerance was excellent clinically and laboratory-wise. This was continued clinical improvement. In January 2007, we decided to stop the program to see what would happen.

In six weeks, her paresthesia and fatigue started to return, so the program was restarted again. By November 15, 2007, she felt well enough to go to China to adopt two more children. On November 18, 2007, all was well with her health and her family. She had moved to Ohio and was homeschooling her children. On June 28, 2007, all was well with her. On May 8, 2008, there were no more complaints. "Brain fog" and fatigue are things of the past. On September 18, 2008, a complete exam was negative in regard to symptoms and findings, and we decided to keep up the program of doxycycline, Flagyl, and Ceftin for another year.

I called her on October 6, 2009, and all was going so well that we decided to continue as we were doing for another year. We stopped all therapy in October 2010.

During this entire period of monitoring, lab work regarding comprehensive metabolic panel, the Epstein-Barr virus, thyroid studies, blood counts, urinalyses, and stool studies were normal. These serial Lyme tests remained negative.

So this is what has happened: We physicians have to realize that the "uncertainty principle" pertains in medicine as well as in physics. We will never know what really happened here, but from my and the patient's vantage point, she has returned to her normal and productive life, and that is what is important (see essay 11).

Patient 11
First Seen: November 29, 2007

This case report is in some detail because it illustrates well the difficulty inherent in treating chronic Lyme disease. The fact that the lab work that has been positive throughout, but positive below the arbitrary limits, convinced three initial well-trained physicians to dismiss the diagnosis.

The patient's disease started in October 2001. At that time, she was bitten by a tick in northern Wisconsin. Three weeks later, she presented herself to an emergency room of a Milwaukee-area hospital with complaints of a pounding heart, headaches, and nausea. She was seen by her internist, who thought she had "a mild viral infection." However, he suspected Lyme disease and ordered "Lyme tests." They revealed anti-Lyme antibodies of 1.42 units and a Western blot of 41 KD IgG. These were interpreted as "normal" by the lab report. He did give her a course of doxycycline (100 mg by mouth for 10 days). This treatment did not help her nausea, weakness, and fatigue, so he referred her to a neurologist. The neurologist agreed that these Lyme tests were negative. He felt the weakness, lower extremity numbness, and her chest pain were due to a panic attack. He did admit her to the hospital for a lumbar puncture which was negative by the usual criteria. The report of levels was apparently not noted by the physicians who ordered it. He also ordered an MRI, but apparently the result never got to him. The report stated:

Prominent, abnormal, deep white matter disease bilaterally. The study is most consistent with a primary demyelinating process such as multiple sclerosis. Other causes of deep white matter disease are possible but are considered less likely, which would include inflammatory and post-infectious processes as well as vasculitic/connective tissue disorders.

With this in hand, I decided to initiate intravenous therapy for chronic Lyme disease. She was seen in St. Mary's Hospital outpatient clinic for a four-week course of ceftriaxone (4 grams per day). There was improvement in all of her symptoms, and they disappeared in six weeks.

This was followed by oral treatment with doxycycline (100 mg by mouth twice a day), erythromycin (500 mg a day by mouth), Flagyl (500 mg a day by mouth), and Ceftin (500 mg by mouth twice a day).

During the past seven years, this patient was closely followed. Her MRI findings improved. In January 2005, a Quest Lyme panel was negative. We stopped the Ceftin and went back to doxycycline, which she tolerated better.

In May 2006, she noted some ataxia and paresthesia. This occurred after she had stopped the doxycycline for a month. This was restarted, and these symptoms disappeared. Also in May 2006, her Quest panel for Bartonella was 1:64 for the first time. We changed the Flagyl to Diflucan for the cystic phase of Borrelia. In June 2006, her symptoms had abated, so we did not opt for another intravenous course of antibiotics. A repeat MRI was "better." She was asymptomatic, but her Babesia titer was positive at 1:128 on the Lyme panel. It is of interest that it took seven years for her Babesia antibody test to surface as positive.

She went back to work full-time. Her Epstein-Barr remained positive, and the Babesia was still 1:128 on the Lyme panel several months later. On a yearly exam on May 1, 2008, she had no complaints and a negative Quest panel.

On a follow-up exam in September 2009, the Quest Lyme panel showed Borrelia antibodies 41 units and Babesia. Even with this lab work, since she had no complaints, we decided just to continue the doxycycline, erythromycin, and Diflucan.

We have here another woman with Lyme disease who had clinical multiple sclerosis. Most important is the fact that her multiple sclerosis findings disappeared after treatment for Lyme disease (see essay 11).

At a follow-up exam on June 7, 2011, she was asymptomatic. For the first time since 2007 she had a positive abdominal reflex in the right upper quadrant, that she previously had not had. Lyme panel now showed Western blot IgM 23 KD. She no longer had Borrelia antibodies nor Babesia antibodies.

Patient 12
First Seen: November 29, 2007

The patient is a sixty-two-year-old retired, male science teacher who spent his summers on a farm in Wisconsin which was in an area known to be infested with deer ticks. At age fifty-five, he developed a progressive syndrome that consisted of generalized muscle cramping and spasm, severe fatigue, difficulty in concentration, neuropathy, pain in both his feet, severe testicular pain, and generalized fasciculation over his torso. (Patient 45 also had severe testicular pain that went away after treatment.)

During the ensuing six years after the onset of the syndrome, all of the symptoms gradually increased until he came to the point that he felt he could no longer function. Visits to many physicians and specialty clinics failed to provide an explanation for this clinical picture.

He searched the Web and came to the conclusion that he might have Lyme disease. He consulted me in this regard, and I agreed that this was a possibility. He agreed to my suggestion that we try an empiric course of intravenous Rocephin (6 grams per day) and oral Flagyl. The Flagyl was given to help his gastrointestinal tract accept the antibiotic and for the theoretical concept that Flagyl might kill forms of Borrelia. He suffered no Herxheimer reaction but made gradual improvement during the initial program.

After the Rocephin, he was maintained on doxycycline (100 mg twice a day) and Flagyl (50 mg given twice per day). His improvement continued, and within weeks he was essentially asymptomatic. The oral treatment was continued for one year. When seen in December 2007, he felt well and was functioning normally. He never consented to have laboratory work.

Patient 13
First Seen: January 24, 2008

This sixty-nine-year-old woman spent time thirty years ago camping all over the country. She was exposed to ticks in the northeast when she camped there. In the twenty-five years during which I have been following her, she has had a litany of diseases that has included chronic gastrointestinal distress, muscle aches and pains, chronic peptic ulcer, joint pain, chronic pancreatitis, and intermittent fever. She became morbidly obese. Most recently, a nodule has been found in her lungs that is being followed with concern. She remembers a tick bite with a bull's-eye rash in 1976. Her Lyme disease panel, done by Quest, showed Lyme antibodies .11 on May 29, 2008, and a Western blot IgG positive band 39.

She has had numerous procedures done by her gastroenterologist. This includes a look at her upper and lower gastrointestinal tracts, of her common duct, and treatment of a chronic peptic ulcer. She has sleep apnea and respiratory distress due to her obesity and surgery for a benign goiter.

Due to her camping history, three years ago I started her on empiric therapy with oral doxycycline (100 mg twice a day) when tolerated. She felt that this has helped control her intermittent fever and her response to her multiple problems. She only takes doxycycline when she can tolerate it, and there has been no evidence of toxicity. She refused further studies regarding Lyme disease.

Does she have chronic Lyme disease? I think she might have, but I have felt that with her multiple problems, all that should be done was to give long-term intermittent oral doxycycline. She has held a full-time job and had an active life during the twenty-five years that I have followed her, until she retired last year.

Patient 14
First Seen: January 09, 2008

In 1992, this highly intelligent and very active registered nurse, when she was fifty years old, suffered a tick bite while in northern Minnesota. A bull's-eye rash was noted, and a blood test was positive for Lyme disease. She was treated for ten days with oral doxycycline in a dosage of 100 mg twice a day.

Several months later, she developed severe fatigue, muscle weakness, and episodes that suggested to some physicians narcolepsy, to others myasthenia gravis. Between 1992 and 2006, when I first saw her, she had consulted "at least" ten physicians, none of whom offered a diagnosis to explain her continuing problems with "brain fog," extreme fatigue, and muscle and joint weakness.

She turned to the Internet and became convinced that she had chronic Lyme disease. After listening to her story, I agreed with her diagnosis and suggested that we treat empirically both the chronic fatigue syndrome and chronic Lyme disease. She agreed because she felt that she had reached "the limit of her endurance."

The program suggested was ceftriaxone to be given for four weeks intravenously at a dosage of 4 grams per day for four weeks, Flagyl (500 mg to be taken by mouth concurrently), and erythromycin (500 mg taken orally four times a day). This was to treat her possible Lyme disease. Concomitantly, she was to be given gamma globulin (4 cc intramuscularly twice a week) during the same four weeks. By mouth, she was to take 2000 mg of Valtrex daily as well as isoprinosine (500 mg four times a day). This was to treat her possible chronic fatigue syndrome and possible fibromyalgia. These were the medications I was using for chronic fatigue in 2006. (Refer to my website, waisbrenclinic. com)

To make a long story short, there was marked improvement in all her symptoms by the end of the four-week period, during which she was receiving antibiotics.

We continued antibiotics by mouth for the next two years as follows: doxycycline (100 mg twice a day), erythromycin (500 mg twice a day), Valtrex (500 mg twice a day), and Flagyl (500 mg once daily).

In 2006, she was taking Ceftin (2 grams per day), Zithromax (2 grams per day), and Nexium. We had to stop the doxycycline because of gastrointestinal effects and had switched her to Ceftin (1 gram per day). She had regained a very active life. We had added Armour thyroid (2 grains twice a day) because of low T_3. This added to her well-being. At her monitoring examination in April 2007, she continued feeling well and had assumed the care of needy children in addition to her three children. She was continuing Ceftin, Zithromax, and Valtrex at her usual doses and was taking Armour thyroid (4 grains per day). Her antibodies against the Epstein-Barr virus were still present. All other monitoring tests were negative. We decided to continue her present program.

When seen on March 26, 2009, she had no symptoms and a complete exam by her personal physician, during which lab studies that were performed were negative. We decided to stop the Ceftin and to continue azithromycin and Valtrex. An MRI ordered at that time showed the "white matter findings" seen in multiple sclerosis and Lyme disease (see essay 11).

By no stretch of the imagination is the case report presented as proof of anything or as a specific suggestion in regard to treatment of any particular patient. Rather, it shows how in desperate situations like this one was, in which the patient had become completely immobile and depressed, an "all-out" attempt at treating all possible problems simultaneously on an empiric basis will sometimes bear fruit. It should be mentioned that her demyelinating symptoms have disappeared. Hopefully, she will eventually consent to another MRI (see essay 11).

Patient 15
First Seen: February 14, 2008

This twenty-two-year-old male Milwaukeean, who comes from a camping family and whose mother had Lyme disease, was seen first on March 23, 2004, and last on December 14, 2008. His complaints were of muscle twitching of his legs and knees. His mother, who had had chronic Lyme disease, made the appointment for me to see him.

On physical examination, the only positive finding was underlying muscle fasciculations of the type seen in amyotrophic lateral sclerosis. His mother and dog had had Lyme disease so, to reassure the mother, I ordered a one-month course of doxycycline and Ceftin. On April 6, 2004, his Quest Lyme panel came back with a screening test only for Bartonella, which suggested at least tick exposure, so I ordered a one-month course of doxycycline, Ceftin, and Flagyl. On May 20, 2004, he said he felt better, so we decided to stop the antibiotics. By September 2004, his screening test for Bartonella was normal but his symptoms of muscle twitching had returned, so we tried another course of doxycycline, Ceftin, and Flagyl. By August 2005, his fasciculation had disappeared but he was again positive on screening test for Bartonella. We stopped medication and scheduled him for an April 2005 appointment. In September 2006, he pronounced himself cured.

When seen a year later, he had some of his original complaints (May 2006). All studies were negative, and he was progressing on his studies for a degree in computer science, so we did not act on his complaints. On August 17, 2006, he had some fasciculation and complaints, but we decided to continue observation. On November 6, 2006, with some more fasciculation and some muscle aches, we decided on another six weeks of doxycycline, Flagyl, and Ketek. In January 2007, he felt better, so the medications were stopped. In February 2007, his complaints returned, so we decided on long-term therapy with doxycycline and Flagyl. Ketek was stopped after a month because his liver enzymes rose. He continued this therapy for a year, until February 2008. When I last saw him in August 2008, he had no complaints and had applied for graduate school. Of course, this case does not prove anything, but all concerned seem satisfied.

Patient 16
First Seen: March 12, 2008

This forty-eight-year-old single woman in the health-care field has been an outdoor camper all her life. She had camped in several tick areas. At age forty-five, she developed a foot drop for which she underwent five spine operations which did not help. In 2005, she developed ataxia, numbness at the bottoms of her both feet, and weakness in both of her legs. She was given Medrol by mouth (36 mg per day), which was tapered to 12 mg per day. A muscle biopsy was equivocal for connective tissue disease. She was assured that she did not have multiple sclerosis but was given no definitive diagnosis.

In 2007, she saw a "Lyme" physician in St. Louis, who made a diagnosis of chronic Lyme disease. He gave her empirically Ceftin, Zithromax, and Flagyl with an apparent clinical response. Studies done by IGeneX revealed negative antibodies for Lyme disease, but there were Western blot bands at 23 to 25 IgG, 31 IgG, 34 IgG, and 41 IgG.

Physical exam revealed ataxia, hyperreflexia, absent abdominal reflexes, and lower extremity muscle weakness. Epstein-Barr titers were elevated at 4.42 IgG. Western blot studies by Quest were negative, as was a lupus panel by Quest. Bartonella, Ehrlichia, and Babesia antibody studies by Quest were negative.

I told the patient that I thought a course of intravenous ceftriaxone, oral erythromycin, and oral Flagyl should be given empirically for four to six weeks. A long conference was held in which she said she would share my opinions with her other "Lyme doctor."

I called her six months later, and she said that her "Lyme doctor" and she were still considering my recommendation. Here we have another case of demyelinating symptoms. She was unwilling to accept my suggestion regarding a lumbar puncture and MRI, and she did not return for follow-up (see essay 11).

Patient 17
Seen: March 19, 2008

This man, who was thirty-three years old when I first saw him in January 2004, was a hunter and fisherman who in August 2003 was bitten by a tick. He developed a bull's-eye rash and a fever and was treated with no response with doxycycline at a dosage of 100 mg twice a day by mouth for ten days. He was referred to me by his doctor in Waukesha, Wisconsin, as a nonresponsive case of Lyme disease. He was suffering from headaches, fatigue, pain, and mental confusion.

On physical examination, he had tender joints but no other positive findings. His Lyme panel by Quest "hit the jackpot." He had seven positive Western blot bands for Borrelia and antibodies against Bartonella and Borrelia by Quest.

He was started, via a PIC line, on intravenous ceftriaxone at a dosage of 6 grams per day. A week later, he broke out in generalized hives. I then switched him, with trepidation, to penicillin G (10 million units a day), given intravenously, along with Flagyl (500 mg per day) on January 27, 2004. There was a clinical response to this. After 20 days, we stopped the IV and continued doxycycline (2 grams a day), Flagyl (500 mg a day), and Zithromax (500 mg twice a day) for his Bartonella. This was continued, with some suspicion of his missing dosages, for eighteen months. He became asymptomatic, although during the first months he noted joint pains when he skipped his doxycycline.

He did not return for follow-up. However, I did call him for a follow-up while writing this report in December 2010. He had stopped all medications in July 2005 and had been entirely well and active since. His Lyme panels by Quest were negative in 2007 and 2008.

His tolerating intravenous penicillin after developing severe hives with ceftriaxone is of particular interest, and I would do the same if presented with the same problem, keeping an EpiPen handy, as we did then, for the possible anaphylaxis.

Patient 18
First Seen: October 2008

This case is presented in some detail because gastrointestinal difficulties that go along with chronic Lyme disease will be familiar to those involved with this disease. They have been designated Bell's palsy of the gut by Dr. Virginia Sherr, a psychiatrist who first noted this syndrome and named it.

This sixty-three-year-old teacher in northern Wisconsin had spent a lifetime in outdoor activities. Her illness started in February 2004 with shoulder pain and explosive diarrhea. Associated with this was "brain fog," fatigue, and weight loss. She suspected Lyme disease and requested studies in this regard, which came back "positive." A course of Biaxin and Ceftin resulted in explosive diarrhea, which may have been partially due to a Herxheimer reaction.

Through a series of doctors, a diagnosis of sprue was made. The succession of doctors she saw were acquainted with sprue disease, and she also saw a series of dietitians. In spite of their efforts, when she presented herself to me, her weight had gone from 105 to 80 pounds, and she was barely able to navigate. She had been assured that she did not have Lyme disease because not enough Western blot bands were "positive" to make this diagnosis. However, just looking at her, one could only conclude that she was at "death's door."

At that time, at the St. Mary's burn center, where I was the internist involved, we had been using hyper alimentation to support patients who could not eat (B. A. Waisbren, "Infection Control and Total Parenteral

Nutrition," archive, *Internal Medicine* 30 [1978]: 175). Accordingly, I felt that the first order of business was to put her bowel at complete rest and to support her with hyper alimentation while we empirically treated her Lyme disease.

The program we decided upon was as follows:

1. Nothing by mouth except sips of water for six weeks.
2. Complete hyper alimentation, which I arranged with a home-health agency, using the system developed at the burn center at St. Mary's Hospital in Milwaukee.
3. Intravenous ceftriaxone at a dosage of 4 grams daily, given by IV push in a PIC line, managed by a home-care agency.
4. Treatment would be monitored by serial studies of blood and electrolytes.

Extensive pretreatment and during-treatment studies failed to establish a diagnosis of sprue. She had low titers of antinuclear antibodies. A biopsy of her small bowel, which was done to study her bowel, showed a lymphocytic infiltration throughout the small-bowel mucosa. A study by IGeneX, which the patient finally agreed to have, showed antibodies against Borrelia and Bartonella.

What follows is the patient's analysis of what happened:

Aspirus home-health workers enabled me to work with my PIC line connecting the food bag and Rocephin easily. I was able to teach during the day, come home at 3:00, connecting Rocephin to the PIC line from a backpack, and this enabled me to do light housework. I then changed connections to the food bag from the backpack to the PIC line. Sleeping: I slept through the night, taking in the nourishment from the food bag. The backpack beeper woke me at 7:00 in the morning. Off refreshed, I went to school. I continued with Rocephin past the initial four weeks, as it was going well and appeared helpful. Each week, the Aspirus home-health worker pleasantly changed my dressings and checked how I was doing, including blood pressure and monitoring lab work. That was in 2005. This is now being written in spring 2008. I feel I beat the Lyme disease.

I continue a gluten-free diet along with the SCD Diet (Specific Carbohydrate Diet), avoiding also a number of foods that were found with lab testing or elimination testing. Recently I found a benefit in taking out all calcium carbonate from what I ingest. This is not a common need for most people, but this was helpful for me. Due to my doctors' work, I also am now on a low-oxalate diet. This diet seems to be needed by some who need a gluten-free diet and has made a huge difference in my digestive tract. Slowly I tried adding some of these listed foods back to my diet, only to have it confirm that I really need them out of my diet. At this time, I do Spirulina and also take a dairy probiotic supplement, Lactobacillus acidophilus. My digestive tract appears to be in the process of healing fully.

I am at work and will continue to work closely with my physicians concerning my gluten-free diet and my other needs. I also consult my dietitians at regular intervals. I am back to cross-country skiing, biking, and walking. I continue to teach, am learning Spanish, and volunteer in my community. I stay away from risks of tick exposure and find safer ways to enjoy the outdoors. My weight has risen to its usual status, which is 110 pounds.

At a follow-up exam in July of 2011, she weighed 110 pounds and had recently, at age 60, taken a 50 mile bike trip. Conclusion: Does this case prove anything? Of course not; however, it might be of interest to those who are engaged in trying to help people with gastrointestinal problems with Lyme disease.

Patient 19
First Seen: April 2008

This woman was sixty-four years of age when I first saw her in April 2008. I had successfully treated her niece for Lyme disease some years before. She had a cottage in Lyme country in northern Wisconsin. She remembered a tick bite in 2003 or 2004 which had been followed by a skin rash and a stiff neck. She began to feel "lousy" shortly thereafter and, up to the time that I saw her, had "brain fog," muscle and joint pains, fatigue, and recurrent skin rashes. In 2006, a physician in northern Wisconsin who treated Lyme disease started her on what he called phased treatment for Lyme disease. He alternated doxycycline and two other antibiotics. One was clarithromycin, and she did not know the name of the other. The physician's philosophy was that he would allow the organisms to recover from the initial antibiotics and then they would be more sensitive when antibiotics were restarted. As I mention later among my essays, I do not believe in this philosophy.

In spite of this program which went on for four years, she came to me with complaints of feeling "lousy," joint pains, muscle pains, recurrent skin rashes, increasing "brain fog," and an irregular heartbeat. She remained on clarithromycin as prescribed by her "previous doctor."

Her Quest panel showed 41 KD IgM and Babesia 1:124. Even before the results were back, I started her on intravenous ceftriaxone (4 grams), clarithromycin (500 mg twice a day), Biaxin (twice a day), Flagyl (500 mg a day), and Valtrex (100 mg twice a day). There was immediate improvement, but it was so slow that after four weeks we increased the dose of ceftriaxone to 6 grams a day. After the six weeks of intravenous therapy, we stopped the intravenous ceftriaxone and continued her on Flagyl, Valtrex, and erythromycin for a few more months.

Since then, she had been in very good health until the fall of 2010, when she developed herpes of her mouth and many of the symptoms of her Lyme disease occurred. Accordingly, we gave her another month of Ceftin, erythromycin, and Flagyl. That seemed to then allow her to continue her job as a substitute gym teacher without further complaints. Her most recent studies show antibodies to Babesia, but she continues to be asymptomatic.

Patient 20
First Seen: May 14, 2008

This is a fifty-three-year-old woman who camped in California yearly from age forty to fifty. In February 2006, she noted atrophy of the muscles in her left hand. The "twitching" of her muscles started in June 2007. A diagnosis of amyotrophic lateral sclerosis was made by Dr. Brooks at the Neurology Clinic at University of Wisconsin Medical School. By the time I saw her on May 14, 2008, her ALS had markedly progressed in spite of the treatment program instituted by Dr. Brooks, which included riluzole (50 mg per day by mouth). By this time, she had generalized muscle weakness, was wheelchair bound, and had involvement of her respiratory muscles. She and her husband had vigorously searched the Internet in an attempt to find some help.

They then found Dr. Rothstein's work which had shown that in animals which had a disease similar to ALS that the glutamate levels were elevated due to a breakdown of a feedback mechanism that regulated the level of this substance. Furthermore, they were aware that under Dr. Rothstein's direction, a double-blind study had been started to see if ceftriaxone, an antibiotic used to treat Lyme disease, which for some reason controlled glutamate intracellular levels in the body, would help ALS.

They contacted a center that was involved in this study. However, they were unable to accept the double-blind method used in this study because they felt that she would die if by chance she was denied ceftriaxone. Since I had published, on my website, my negative feelings about double-blind studies being done on dying patients who might be helped by the drug being used in a study, they presented themselves with the request that I orchestrate a program that would give her high doses of ceftriaxone on an open basis. They were able to convince their insurance company to go along with treatment with 6 grams of ceftriaxone given daily intravenously by a home-care agency. They were fully cognizant of the fact that this program would be strictly empiric.

The following program was started:

1. Ceftriaxone (2 grams) was given intravenously in the outpatient department of St. Mary's Hospital.
2. Then, since it was tolerated, it was arrange for her to have 6 grams of ceftriaxone daily through a PIC line at home.

She was also to take Flagyl (500 mg twice a day by mouth). The program was to be monitored by a basic metabolic panel, urinalysis, and a complete blood count weekly. A detailed informed consent was signed by the patient and her husband.

Toleration of the program was excellent, but in spite of it, her disease continued to worsen. The treatment was discontinued after two months, and she died of respiratory failure in August 2008.

The only positive in this case was that it gave the patient some hope and it demonstrated, as I found repeatedly in the past, that ceftriaxone given intravenously at a dose of 6 grams per day is well tolerated clinically if followed by laboratory monitoring. The liver enzyme elevation that we have seen in the past did not occur. A Lyme panel done by Quest was negative for Borrelia, Bartonella, Ehrlichia, and Babesia.

Patient 21
First Seen: May 29, 2008

This thirty-six-year-old woman had tick exposure in Wisconsin in mid-2008. Following this, she began to feel lousy, had "brain fog," ankle swelling, and extreme fatigue. She saw her physician on April 21, 2008, and he diagnosed chronic Lyme disease on the basis of her exposure, blood tests positive for B. burgdorferi antibodies, and Western blot bands positive at 23 KN IgM, 41 KD IgM. She was given 100 mg of doxycycline three times a day for three weeks. She could not tolerate the doxycycline, so she discontinued it for two weeks. All of her symptoms continued.

I repeated the laboratory tests, and by the same laboratory her Borrelia antibodies were negative, the Western blot findings were negative. Tests for Babesia and Ehrlichia were negative (the ordered test for Bartonella was not done). As so often happens with my cases of Lyme disease, the titer for Epstein-Barr virus was positive. A screening test for lupus and other autoimmune diseases was negative (Quest).

I concurred with the diagnosis of Lyme disease and suggested the following treatment by the oral route: penicillin G (4 grams per day by mouth), azithromycin (500 mg by mouth twice a day), Flagyl (500 mg by mouth daily), and Valtrex (1000 mg twice a day by mouth).

If the regimen did not help "brain fog," fatigue, and muscle pain in three weeks, or if it was not tolerated, we would try four to six weeks of intravenous ceftriaxone with antibiotics covering Bartonella. We would continue the Valtrex, add intramuscular gamma globulin for the fatigue, and continue Diflucan or Flagyl for the cystic phase of Borrelia.

She was seen three weeks later. She had started the oral program, developed C. difficile/diarrhea, and had stopped the antibiotics. Her diarrhea was improving with probiotics. We decided to wait a month before reconsidering intravenous ceftriaxone.

She did not keep her next appointment, and as of this date, October 25, 2009, I have not been able to get in touch with her for follow-up.

This case reveals that "you can't win them all" and that many cases of chronic Lyme disease present with multiple problems.

Patient 22
First seen: June 5, 2008

This fifty-nine-year-old, highly intelligent, hyperactive, highly persuasive woman was bitten by a tick in 1993 and developed a rash characteristic of Lyme disease. She was kind enough to write me her history which, as one can see, resulted in reams of medical records.

Elements of her self-written medical history follow:

In 1995, while living in the East and leading a very productive and active life, I "think" I was bitten by a tick. I began having trouble in concentrating and collecting my thoughts. I then began to have severe fatigue and muscle weakness. The doctors in the East that I saw could not explain my generalized decline in regard to cognition, locomotion, energy, muscle weakness, and the beginning of gradual weight gain, which went from me being plump to extreme obesity. In desperation, I moved to my hometown in the Midwest. During the next two years I became disabled to the point that I had to be "spoon-fed" by my mother. I saw 20 doctors, none of whom seemed to be able to help me. One bright spot was when, because of a respiratory infection, I was given an antibiotic by a relative who was a physician. For several weeks, while taking the antibiotic, I felt better.

Finally, after two horrific years of illness, I consulted an infectious disease specialist in Kansas City. He made the diagnosis of chronic Lyme disease and sequentially over the next year treated me with Biaxin (500 mg twice a day) and ceftriaxone (3 grams a day intravenous), which was stopped because, as I think now, I had a Herxheimer reaction—a known complication of ceftriaxone therapy. During the years between 2005 and

2007, during which I was being treated with antibiotics, I first seemed to be responding, but then my condition worsened. I could not hold down food. My cognition got worse, I developed generalized muscle and joint pains, and I became wheelchair bound. My gastrointestinal system "recoiled," and I frequently vomited but continued to gain weight.

I first consulted Dr. Waisbren on June 5, 2008, with all of the above problems.

The above is what I heard carefully explained on June 5, 2008. Physical examination revealed only an obese woman with some joint and muscle tenderness. She had brought along recent laboratory results that only seemed to indicate that she was "in good shape for the shape that she was in." She did not have with her the test results for Lyme disease, which apparently had been somewhat equivocal.

Faced with her almost-complete immobility and the length of her illness, I decided to make a clinical diagnosis of chronic Lyme disease with probable related tick diseases and the gastrointestinal disease described by Dr. Virginia Sherr as "Bell's palsy of the gut."

I discussed with her my opinion that the severity of her condition suggested to me that it would be reasonable to empirically treat all the manifestations of Lyme disease, with which I had become familiar, with maximum tolerated doses of all modalities and maneuvers that might help her. She agreed with and understood the rationales of the elements of the program I proposed.

The elements proposed were as follows:

1. A long-term intravenous program done through a PIC line of 4 grams of ceftriaxone given daily for a five-day week.
2. Oral Ceftin (500 mg by mouth twice a day).
3. Erythromycin (500 mg by mouth twice a day) for presumed Bartonella.
4. Diflucan for the cystic form of Borrelia.
5. Valtrex (1000 mg by mouth twice a day) for co infection with the Epstein-Barr virus.
6. Gamma globulin (4 cc intramuscularly weekly) for blocking antibodies against the autoimmune aspect of chronic Lyme disease.

7. Reduce oral intake of food to a minimum and substitute hyper alimentation given through the PIC line to rest her gut. The hyper alimentation protocol was one I used on burn patients for many years and included multiple vitamins to the point of toleration. She was to use hyper alimentation when she felt that her gastrointestinal tract needed a rest. She has continued this program off and on based on toleration to the present.

All of this would be instituted with the help of Coram HealthCare Agency, a national agency specializing in home-care intravenous therapy.

We agreed that anything we did that seemed to impinge on her quality of life would be stopped. Monitoring of her basic metabolic panel and hematologic picture would be done weekly, biweekly, and then monthly.

I last saw this patient for follow-up in September 2010 and in February 2011. She initiated the program I suggested but kept it at a level that did not impinge on her daily activities. This included hyper alimentation and intravenous ceftriaxone. As of February 2011, she was holding her own and is contemplating surgery for her morbid obesity. I interpret this care as a possible satisfactory program for a patient with chronic Lyme disease and Bell's palsy of the gut, as described by Dr. Sherr. She continues on intermittent intravenous ceftriaxone, at her insistence. She is living an active, productive life. All in all, she feels she has been helped. (Although, currently in September 2011, I think that the treatments for babesia and bartonella that I now use in recalcitrant cases might be in order.

Patient 23
First Seen: July 17, 2008

This forty-eight-year-old landscape gardener, who has had daily exposure to ticks, was seen first on July 17, 2008. For the past three years, he had had concentration problems, joint pain, fatigue, weight loss, and neck pain. His wife had had Lyme disease before he was sick, and she had been treated with antibiotics.

Physical exam revealed some joint tenderness but was otherwise essentially normal. He had never been sick before 2005, when his syndrome started. He had seen a neurologist, who assured him that he did not have multiple sclerosis. His laboratory studies by Quest were negative, but IGeneX found antibodies against Borrelia 1:80, Bartonella 1:20, and Western blot IgM 23–25, IgG 20, 31, 34, 41, 83.

I agreed with the diagnosis of chronic Lyme disease that the patient had come up with. I saw him on May 12, 2008; September 4, 2008; and January 8, 2009. I decided on a sequential attempt to try to help him. First, we tried doxycycline (100 mg three times a day), erythromycin (500 mg three times a day), and Flagyl (500 mg a day). When this helped a bit but did not alleviate the high level of fatigue, we then tried Valtrex (1000 mg three times a day) and gamma globulin (4 cc twice a week for four weeks) to treat his Epstein-Barr infestation.

The gamma globulin was to provide blocking antibodies to mute the autoimmunity that accompanies chronic Lyme disease. When the clinical response, if any, was very little, I suggested an eight-week course of intravenous ceftriaxone, Ketek (400 mg by mouth twice a day),

Diflucan (200 mg twice a week). The Ketek was to be held the days he received Diflucan because of difficulties that occur when the drugs are taken together.

The patient investigated his third-party coverage for this program, and I received the following letter on January 15, 2009. At that point, I thought it best that he try the physician who he mentioned in his letter.

His price investigation shows dilemmas which chronic Lyme disease patients face:

Dear Dr. Waisbren:

I'm writing to you to give you an update on my IV treatments. Yesterday I found out it would cost $321 a day for materials. My insurance said they would pay $310 a day, but they would use my coverage for the hospital stay ($300 a day) to cover the Rocephin and materials. This seems a little odd to do it this way, so I need to confirm.

Today I contacted a national drug store because they also do this service. Their price is ($297) and they may be contacting you. So I did postpone the PIC line for now as I must find out for sure if I can afford all of this. There will be additional costs for in-home nurses and lab work.

I do appreciate all that you have done so far. If this becomes too costly, I may have to stick with the oral antibiotics. My mother's friend is currently being treated for Lyme's by a Lyme-literate doctor in Fond du Lac. Her first antibiotics are as follows: Tindamax (500 mg—1 capsule 3 times daily), Omnicef (300 mg—2 capsules in the morning), Biaxin XL (500 mg—2 capsules at suppertime). These are all different than what I've tried so far so maybe I'd get good results with the change. I know you want me to get better so maybe it is worth a try, if you agree.

While I wait to see if the pharmacy is any more affordable, could you make out prescriptions for these antibiotics for 6–8 weeks, and I could pick them up later today. Thank you for all you have done.

I told the patient that I could not make out the prescriptions that he requested since I had no experience with them, and I have not seen or heard from him since.

Patient 24
First Seen: August 28, 2008

Note: I am not asking the reader to accept this case as Lyme disease. It is being included to fulfill the inclusive nature of this report. At the least it illustrates the diagnostic difficulties in separating syndromes such as chronic fatigue, Lyme disease, and anxiety, and how treating *possibilities*, even remote, sometimes pay off clinically.

The patient is a thirty-six-year-old Wisconsinite who moved to Eagle River, Wisconsin. I first saw her on August 28, 2008, at age twenty-two. She had been exposed to ticks. She brought along a three-page typed review of her symptoms. Her illness started approximately in 2001, when after a second pregnancy she noted extreme fatigue, sinus difficulties, and insomnia. Her father had developed narcolepsy, and she began to note periods of intermittent extreme sleepiness during the day. She had seen a succession of doctors and had a complete workup at a major Wisconsin clinic, to no avail in regard to diagnosis or treatment of her extreme fatigue, daylight sleepiness, and insomnia. The most popular diagnosis was depression and anxiety. By August 28, 2008, she was nonfunctioning in regard to taking care of her two young children.

She had always been in excellent health before the onset of her symptoms. She had a sleep study which was said to be positive and had tried Ambien, which did not solve her problems. Physical examination was negative. Initial laboratory findings revealed a Western blot IgM positive at 41 (Quest), a Western blot IgG of 44, Epstein-Barr 4.31, normal thyroid studies, and a negative Quest screen for autoimmunity. During one of her workups, her spleen was enlarged.

The positive findings then were insomnia, fatigue, a high titer of the Epstein-Barr virus, episodes of sleepiness during the day, and Western blot from Quests, positive at 41 and 43. Faced with a completely nonfunctioning young woman, I decided to treat sequentially the findings on an empiric basis. I started with Armour thyroid (4 grains daily). There was no clinical response between August 28, 2008, and April 16, 2009. I then decided on empiric treatment for Lyme disease based on her symptoms and the Western blot IgM 41 and IgG 44 by Quest. She was given Ketek (400 mg twice a day), doxycycline (100 mg twice a day), and Flagyl (300 mg a day). I also began empiric treatment of narcolepsy, which consisted of Provigil to take at sleepy times and up to twice a day. I stopped the Valtrex which I had prescribed for the Epstein-Barr virus.

I then saw her on May 14, 2009. There had been definite improvement in all spheres. She said, "You gave me my life back."

On August 6, 2009, improvement had continued, and she was living a normal life and had needed Provigil only rarely. At that time, a screening lupus test (Quest) showed an ANA titer of 1:40; the Western blot 41 positively had disappeared. The test for tick-related disease remained negative. An MRI of the brain was normal.

On November 4, 2009, she felt that she had been "cured" and the Western blot of 41 had not returned, nor were there signs of a tick-related disease.

I decided to continue the Lyme treatment for another six months and discontinued the Provigil. A note from the patient said, "I am feeling the best I have in six years."

Note: I will leave it up to the reader to interpret this case.

Patient 25
First Seen: September 10, 2008

On July 13, 2008, this patient, thirty-five years of age, while bicycling in Lyme country in Wisconsin, sustained a tick bite on his neck. Nine days later, he noted a low-grade fever, joint aches, sore neck, and pain in his testicles. He developed a rash on both legs. On August 9, 2008, he went to his doctor, who made a diagnosis of Lyme disease and also prescribed doxycycline (100 mg) to be taken by mouth for three weeks. The rash disappeared in several days. On September 1, 2008, the rash reappeared, and he developed night sweats and twitching of his neck muscles. He noted an irregular heartbeat.

I saw him on September 10, 2008. His physical exam was essentially negative, but he did have a faint erythematous rash over his thorax. His laboratory studies, done by Quest, were negative for Bartonella, Babesia, and Ehrlichia; and positive for Borrelia (Lyme disease). His Western blot (Quest) was positive for bands 58, 41, 39, 23 KDA (IgM).

The clinical diagnosis seemed apparent, so I prescribed Ceftin (500 mg by mouth three times per day), Flagyl (500 mg once daily), doxycycline (100 mg twice a day), and erythromycin (500 mg by mouth twice a day).

When seen on November 13, 2008, he was essentially asymptomatic and had tolerated the therapeutic program well. We decided to continue the oral medications for another year.

When he was seen in January 2009, he was asymptomatic, so treatment was discontinued. He said he would come in on an as-needed basis.

Patient 26
First Seen: September 18, 2008

This forty-year-old male was first seen by me in September 2008. History revealed that as an outdoorsman, he had had numerous exposures to ticks in northern Illinois and Wisconsin. His health had always been excellent, and he had no significant past medical history or family history.

He first noticed that he had a health problem in January 2007. At that time, he started to develop extreme fatigue, "brain fog," and muscle and joint pain. His ability to continue daily workouts in the gym began to wane. He gradually developed gastrointestinal symptoms consisting of abdominal pain and diarrhea.

In order to obtain an explanation for the above problems, all of which had increased during the period from January 2007 to September 2008, he had consulted ten physicians, most of whom were specialists in their fields. Included among them were gastroenterologists, rheumatologists, a specialist in infectious diseases, psychiatrists, and physiotherapists. All performed studies suggested by their special interests, and none seemed to be able to make a definitive diagnosis. Most felt that he was depressed, and he had received two antidepressants which did not help him. The infectious disease doctor considered Lyme disease and gave him a short course of doxycycline. He discontinued it when a blood test came back "negative."

The patient studied the Internet and came to the conclusion that he may have Lyme disease. He came to me for information and possible treatment for this disease because, as he put it, "I seem to be coming to an end of my rope."

After hearing his story and going over the many studies that had been done, I concluded that because of his exposure and the ruling out of many diseases by the various specialists that he had seen, it would be reasonable to empirically treat him for Lyme disease even before the laboratory studies came back. His symptom complex at that time consisted of extreme fatigue, muscle weakness, a strange rash of strip-like lesions over his chest and under his arms, some dizziness, "brain fog," and muscle tightness. (A dermatologist had not been able to diagnose the rash which subsequently I found out was characteristic of that found in bartonellosis, which we now feel he had.) He had had laboratory work done on his own initiative by the IGeneX Lab in California that, when I obtained it, confirmed a positive antibody test for Lyme disease and Western blot studies, which I have found often are present in Lyme disease. Interestingly, studies I ordered from the Quest Laboratory were all "negative" for Lyme disease.

He agreed to an empiric trial of antibiotics for Lyme disease, and I started him on doxycycline (100 mg twice a day), erythromycin (500 mg twice a day), and Flagyl (500 mg daily). His gastrointestinal problems flared up so intensely after ten days that we had to stop all antibiotics.

I then explained to him that because of his initial intolerance to antibiotics given by mouth and by his ongoing sprue-like symptoms (this disease had been suggested by several of his gastroenterologists who prescribed a gluten-free diet), I thought it would be reasonable to put his bowel at rest for six weeks by a nothing-by-mouth program, hyper alimentation, and to place him on antibiotics given intravenously at the same time. This strategy I had found effective in a case very similar to his (reported on my website and in the literature, case 18 in this series).

Unfortunately at this time, his insurance company that had paid for his two years of testing and consultations "kicked up its heels" and decided not to give any more coverage. Consequently, for financial and family reasons, the patient decided to move with his wife to the East to be nearer his family.

He asked me to refer him to a doctor interested and knowledgeable about Lyme disease. Through the Internet, I decided to refer him to Dr.

Virginia Sherr, who had a particular interest in gastrointestinal problems associated with chronic Lyme disease. Dr. Sherr kindly consented to see him, and she agreed with the diagnosis and added to it by getting a "Fry" test which showed presumed Bartonella organisms invading the patient's red cells. Her diagnosis was neuro- and gastric-bartonellosis and Lyme disease. She referred the patient to a Lyme-sophisticated physician in her area. During the period between March 2009 and July 2009, while being treated by this physician, he suffered a severe allergic reaction to Ceftin and had an indifferent response to intramuscular drugs prescribed by the "Lyme" specialists.

When I last heard from the patient in April 2009, he still was suffering from gastrointestinal, muscular, energy, and mentation problems. In addition, he had developed generalized urticaria. I believe that the next step should have been gamma globulin, nothing by mouth for a month of hyper alimentation, and gentamicin intramuscularly for Bartonella which, because of his rash, I think are the main offending organisms. Financial problems and insurance now have him essentially stuck in regard to further treatment. I am inclined to think at this point the bartonellosis (Fry test), which is in some cases relatively antibiotic resistant, is the main culprit here. Review of the literature regarding bartonellosis suggests that amino glycosides and rifampicin should be tried next in recalcitrant bartonellosis.

This patient illustrates most of the problems inherent in patients with Lyme disease and accompanying complications getting state-of-the-art treatment for this condition. They are:

1. Unfamiliarity with this disease by many subspecialists.
2. Very prestigious laboratories' reports of negative findings when positive findings exist.
3. A stone wall regarding payment for treatments by many insurance companies.
4. The fact that because of present problems in Lyme disease treatments, the patient has been unable to receive beneficial antibiotics for his bartonellosis (Fry test) and autoimmunity (gamma globulin).

At this point (February 2011), I think that chronic bartonellosis is probably an important factor in nonresponsive chronic Lyme disease. As shown by studies done in Peru, where bartonellosis is endemic, it is sometimes resistant to all antibiotics except bactericidal gentamicin (an amino glycoside) and rifampicin. I believe that these two drugs might be helpful to him, but unfortunately I have lost contact with him.

Patient 27
First Seen: November 2, 2008

This seventy-two-year-old woman suffered an "inflamed" tick bite in Rhinelander, Wisconsin, in late September 2008. Three weeks later, her left knee swelled up and became painful. She saw her physician, who prescribed Ceftin and did a Lyme test. He gave her an injection of "cortisone" into her knee. There was no improvement in the knee pain, and her wrist began to hurt and become swollen. A month later, she was seen again by the same physician. He noted in her chart that the Lyme disease test was "positive" and prescribed another course of Ceftin by mouth.

When there continued to be knee and wrist pain and a feeling of being "unwell," she presented herself to me on November 2, 2008. Her Western blot test was positive at 41 KD, and she had an ANA titer of 1:40. Because of the history and the Western blot, I decided to treat her for Lyme disease even though the Quest antibody and associated infection titers were negative. Her Epstein-Barr titer was positive. (As will be seen in other cases, the Epstein-Barr virus may be a candidate for a co infection associated with Lyme disease.)

After a careful discussion in which we emphasized that we were treating as a possible case of Lyme disease, she was started by mouth on doxycycline (100 mg twice a day), Ketek (400 mg twice a day), and Flagyl (500 mg daily).

When seen in mid-January 2009, her complaints had narrowed to just knee pain, and she felt much better clinically. She declined further laboratory studies since her Western blot 41 KD and original antibody studies had become normal.

She continued the oral program for a total of five months and then was lost to follow-up. I would have liked to see if her antinuclear antibody titers had returned to normal. If so, it would add further credence to the thought that treatment of Lyme disease might help the autoimmune aspects of this disease.

Patient 28
First Seen: November 13, 2008

This sixty-seven-year-old Milwaukeean had documented Lyme disease in 1994. It was treated with ceftriaxone in an intravenous dose of 4 grams per day for three weeks. It was followed by weakness of her left leg and chronic gastrointestinal disease that baffled a series of physicians who did multiple diagnostic tests over the next decade.

In July 2008, she had developed a "florid morbilliform" eruption which disappeared in four days. "Lyme tests" by her dermatologist were negative. She had continued rashes, and her cardiologist, after reviewing her history, referred her to me with the question, "Could her rash and years of gastrointestinal difficulties be due to chronic Lyme disease?" My examination revealed weakness of her left leg and ongoing complaints of chronic gastrointestinal problems. The Quest screening tests revealed only a Western blot of IgG 41. She was reluctant to have a small-bowel biopsy, to see if there was the lymphocytic infiltration I have seen in Lyme Bell's palsy of the gut, and more intensive Lyme tests. I did not blame her because in ten years she had been "lymed out." Accordingly, we decided on an empiric course of oral penicillin (500 mg by mouth twice a day). This had the best possibility of not causing gastrointestinal problems.

I saw her in follow-up three months later. She had tolerated the oral penicillin well and felt that it might have helped her. On August 15, 2009, she reported that she was tolerating 500 mg of penicillin G per day and that she would like to continue it. For the first time, she did show antibodies against Borrelia. Her gastrointestinal problems were fairly quiescent but still present.

The appearance of anti-Borrelia antibodies makes the diagnosis of chronic Lyme disease with Bell's palsy of the gut more possible. We are continuing the oral penicillin.

Patient 29
First Seen: November 10, 2008

This thirty-nine-year-old brilliant computer programmer presented himself on November 10, 2008 based on his Internet study. As is my practice, I asked him, "How can I help you?" His reply was, "Treat my Lyme disease." Somewhat taken aback, I said, "I thought I was the diagnostician, but what is your story?" He was kind enough to write up his story:

I have been exposed to ticks because I am an avid bike rider in the woods. In mid-April 2008, something bit the back of my hand. The next day, the area was red, tender, and swollen. Over a period of the next few weeks, I felt flu-like, developed numbness and tingling over my face and arms, and photophobia [he knew what this was]. In addition, the left side of my face was tingling and drooped.

I am embarrassed to tell you how many doctors I have consulted. They've spent thousands of dollars on my workups that included an MRI of my head and a spinal tap. They thought my problem was all in my "head."

Finally, I turned to the Internet and based upon what I found, I decided I'd better see you for treatment of the Lyme disease that I concluded I had. I do not want any more tests; I just want treatment.

I told him that what he said seemed logical and asked if he would at least let me examine him first and get a Lyme panel. He agreed, and my examination revealed drooping of the left side of his face and, to my surprise, fasciculations along his upper extremities. The remainder of the examination was negative.

In spite of the fact that his Lyme panel was negative, his history was so persuasive that we agreed upon the following plan. We would do laboratory work and then start him on oral treatment for Lyme disease. If there was no response, we would consider other options, which include more precise studies for Lyme disease, spinal fluid glutamate levels for amyotrophic lateral sclerosis, given his fasciculations which are characteristic of that disease, and as a last resort, intravenous therapy for Lyme disease. He was reassured when I told him that this was not in his mind and that he did not need the tranquilizers suggested by other physicians.

He was started on doxycycline (100 mg twice a day by mouth), Ketek (400 mg twice a day by mouth), oral penicillin (500 mg twice a day), and Flagyl (500 mg daily). The response of his fatigue, paresthesia, myalgia, and fasciculations was so good that we continued these medications until October 2008. At that time, he discontinued medications to see what would happen. What happened was that the symptoms recurred. After three weeks, he resumed his original therapy. For the next two weeks, he felt worse and had night sweats and fever. Following this, he again began to feel very well, and he continued the antibiotic program until I saw him one year later, in October 2009. He had been completely asymptomatic during the previous year.

We both felt that the discomfort after the reinstitution of the antibiotics was due to a Herxheimer reaction, which of course is seen after treatment of chronic Lyme disease. It is of interest that the Bell's palsy symptoms of his left face had reappeared when he stopped therapy, only to resolve after restarting his original therapy. There was no sign of left-face drooping or fasciculations on the November 2010 examination.

Summary: This was a thirty-nine-year-old man who made his own diagnosis based on readings from the Internet. He had Bell's palsy and other signs of central nervous system involvement (e.g., ataxia and fasciculations of the type found in amyotrophic lateral sclerosis). He responded to two courses of oral antibiotics. The second was given when his symptoms returned after the first course was stopped. He had a probable Herxheimer reaction after the antibiotics were resumed, and then became asymptomatic. He continued the oral antibiotics for one year. His neurologic exam returned to normal, and he was asymptomatic. He refused further studies, stopped the antibiotics, and has remained without symptoms. While his neurologic symptoms were suspicious for demyelination, they were *not* suggestive enough to include this diagnosis in this series.

Patient 30
First Seen: February 19, 2009

This fifty-nine-year-old English teacher and outdoors woman was in excellent health until 1992, when she developed ataxia. Multiple sclerosis was suspected, and an MRI showed the white spots characteristic of this disease as well as with multiple sclerosis (see essay 11). She was given "antibiotic treatment" for tinnitus which seemed to help. Studies for Lyme disease showed Western blot results considered diagnostic for Lyme disease.

She had led backpack trips for many years on both coasts. She remembered a "bull's-eye" rash in 1991, when camping on the beach in Mendocino, California.

She still had neurologic symptoms in 1995 and consulted a group of doctors known to be interested in Lyme disease. On their advice, she started an antibiotic course that included intramuscular penicillin.

In 1999 she consulted Dr. Chaney regarding her Lyme disease, and he gave her two weeks of intravenous antibiotic therapy. There was a definite clinical response.

In 2001, she received ten days of hyperbaric oxygen therapy for Lyme disease. In April 2008, all blood tests for Lyme disease were "good," although she still felt that she had a chronic disease that was "sapping" her strength. In October 2008, she was given doxycycline (100 mg five times a day), erythromycin (500 mg twice a day), and Septra (2 grams per day).

I first saw her on February 19, 2009. She related her story and gave me a copy of the above information. On physical exam, she had right-sided weakness, absent abdominal reflexes, and a staggering gait. Laboratory exam showed a high titer against cytomegalovirus 13.2, Lyme antibody titer of 0.23, and a high titer against the Epstein-Barr virus. Studies for co-infections with tick exposure were all negative.

I felt that this was another case of multiple sclerosis associated with chronic Lyme disease (see essay 11). I suggested a course of intravenous ceftriaxone to be followed by daily Copaxone. I arranged for a PIC line to be placed here in Milwaukee, and she went on her planned trip to California, where she went after accepting my suggestion that she use the Pic line for her IV therapy of the ceftriaxone and oral erythromycin. She had assumed the Walgreens Company in California, where she teaches English, would cover the intravenous treatment. They refused based on the Infectious Disease Society's guidelines, so she obtained the I.V. ceftriaxone in Mexico and had the prescriptions for erythromycin and diflucan filled in California.

During a follow-up conversation I had with her in December 2010, she had taken another course of intravenous ceftriaxone which she had obtained in Mexico. She had taken my suggestion that she take Copaxone (30 mg a day intramuscularly) for multiple sclerosis. She is taking gamma globulin intramuscularly and is deciding for herself when she needs more. She also has been able to arrange (I know not how) courses of intravenous ceftriaxone several times in the interim.

She has continued to function as an English teacher, although she still has ataxia and paresthesia. This is another case of demyelination accompanying chronic Lyme disease (see essay 11).

Patient 31
First Seen: March 5, 2009

This woman brought with her a documented history of chronic Lyme disease of fifteen years' duration. There is an associated bipolar component, I think. All of this came out in a two-and-a-half-hour session. She had, in addition to "fatigue," weakness, muscle pain, and gastrointestinal symptoms, ataxia and hyperreflexia. In view of this, I decided that she had enough consultation and studies to justify a "full-court press" of her Lyme disease and possible demyelinating disease. She had not done as well as hoped for on a previous course of intravenous ceftriaxone. I gave her prescriptions for the following:

1. Gamma globulin (4 cc weekly)—for blocking antibodies against antimyelin antibodies.
2. Diflucan (200 mg each day) for the cystic phase of Borrelia.
3. Valtrex (1000 mg twice a day) for Epstein-Barr co infection.
4. Armour thyroid or Synthroid (75 mg per day).
5. Ketek (400 mg by mouth twice a day).
6. Oral penicillin (2 grams three times a day).
7. Copaxone (30 mg subcutaneously daily).

My plan was to institute intravenous therapy if the oral program and a more intensive oral program that I gave her did not help.

In my own mind, I am not sure whether this vibrant woman has what I call narcissistic Lyme disease, in which a patient falls in love with their disease, or indeed has chronic Lyme disease with demyelination.

She said that she would run this program by her "Lyme doctor." I contacted her in April 2010. She said she still was taking the matter under advisement. I have not heard from her since. This case is included to meet my sequential case requirement for this book.

Patient 32
First Seen: March 12, 2009

This sixty-two-year-old Latino woman was first seen on March 12, 2009. She had been chronically ill for thirty years, but had courageously done factory work until mid-2009. Her past history included hepatitis C which had been extensively treated to the point that her viral load for hepatitis C was negative. She had lived in a tick-infested area of Texas until 1992. Her lifestyle had been to work eight hours in a factory and go home to bed, where she stayed the rest of the time. Her daughter, a practical nurse, heard a lecture about chronic Lyme disease while at a convention in California, and concluded that her mother's many years of fever, weakness, anemia, and joint and muscle pain were due to Lyme disease. She came to see me, with her daughter from her home in Indianapolis, in March 2007 with this diagnosis. She had had tick exposure in Texas, where she had lived until she became ill in 1992, when she moved to Indianapolis.

Her physical examination revealed a chronically ill woman with slight fever, muscle weakness, and joint pain. Quest panel only revealed antibodies for Bartonella. An IGeneX study found Borrelia antibodies at 1:16.

Since the patient and her family strongly felt that she was on a path to death, we decided to try an empiric oral course of treatment for Lyme disease and the Epstein-Barr virus which we had found is usually present in chronic Lyme disease.

She was started on by-mouth Ceftin (500 mg three times a day), erythromycin (500 mg three times a day), Diflucan (200 mg daily), and 4 ml of gamma globulin given twice a week. The pills were spaced throughout the day.

There has been a slow but definite response noted the three times I have seen her since. Her hemogram normalized; her liver function remained the same; and her fever, weakness, and joint and muscle pain disappeared. Her Western blot 41 IgG and IgM and Bartonella titer stayed the same. According to her family, she has gone from complete invalid to essential wellness.

Patient 33
First Seen: April 2, 2009

This case is a prime example of "mother knows best." This patient was seen first on April 2, 2009. His story is as follows: He had been exposed to ticks in July 2007. He was a participant in gymnastics and was a member of a championship team. In August 2007, he developed fever, conjunctivitis, and bronchitis. He was treated, apparently successfully, with antibiotics.

However, one month later he developed a syndrome which included fever, episodes of "brain fog," muscle and joint aches, constant headaches, and skin rashes. In February 2008, he had a seizure. A CT scan and EEG were negative. He was then given a ten-day course of clarithromycin, which did not alleviate the fever. In January 2009, his ability as a gymnast began to deteriorate because of balance problems. His schoolwork deteriorated as well, as did his energy level.

His mother, a highly trained psychiatric social worker, had him see a series of doctors, who were unable to make a diagnosis. A Lyme test was said to be negative. After she mounted a search on the Internet, she became concerned that he had Lyme disease. Through the Internet, she found me. The history of tick exposure, "brain fog," loss of coordination, muscle and joint pains, recurrent rashes, and severe headaches certainly was suggestive of chronic Lyme disease.

The examination showed borderline ataxia, hyperactive reflexes, and absent abdominal reflexes. Accordingly, I started him by mouth on doxycycline (100 mg twice a day), Ceftin (500 mg twice a day), Ketek (400 mg twice a day), and Flagyl (500 mg daily).

The Lyme panel by Quest showed IgG bands of the Western blot of 25 KD and 41 KD. Antibodies against Ehrlichia were positive, as were antibodies against Borrelia and Epstein-Barr virus. These were all included in the Quest Lyme panel.

When seen on May 18, 2009, both his mother and the patient felt that he had improved a great deal but that he still had "a long way to go." The most striking improvement was in his constant headaches. I then added intramuscular gamma globulin (2 ml twice weekly).

When seen on July 18, 2009, the improvement had continued and a decision was made to continue therapy. The Western blots from April 2, 2009, were negative, as was the antibodies against Ehrlichia and Borrelia. The mother convinced me to stop all medications in November 2009. When seen on April 20, 2010, the patient had grown two inches, had regained his gymnastics skills, no longer had fever or "brain fog," and was doing extremely well at school.

Summary: This is a clinical case of chronic Lyme disease with some neurologic aspects that clinically responded to oral antibiotic therapy and gamma globulin. He had regained abdominal reflexes and balance. The Western blot to Lyme disease and antibodies to Ehrlichia and Borrelia had disappeared. This is the tenth case of central nervous symptoms with presumed Lyme disease. The symptoms disappeared after treatment (see essay 11).

Patient 34
First Seen: April 9, 2009

This sixty-two-year-old northern Alaskan patient wrote up his case so well that I use his written summary in this series.

In the spring of 2000, on the southern Oregon coast, I developed a tick rash that lasted three to four months. At the time, I thought that Lyme disease was confined to the Upper Midwest and the Northeast. There were other reasons: the tick did not quite match the deer ticks I was used to, and the rash was solid—both observations inconsistent with my notions of Lyme. I dismissed it as an allergic reaction and put it out of my mind.

In the immediate years following, I experienced a number of symptoms I now know to be consistent with Lyme disease: flu-like illnesses which lasted well over a month; extended periods of night sweats; episodes of painful swallowing; dizziness; leg cramps; jaw pain; unnatural anxiety; and extended periods of deep fatigue, followed by long remissions. General blood tests (including thyroid checks for the night sweats) revealed nothing.

In 2004, I developed periods of chronic diarrhea, which would last several months, then remit for long periods. A colonoscopy revealed nothing. About that time, I experienced incapacitating episodes of back pain, as well as transient carpal tunnel–like pains in my wrists and middle fingers. I also experienced the first episode affecting the eyes, with pinkening of one eye and the development of floaters. My tinnitus may have begun about that time. During my three worst diarrheal episodes, I developed extensive rashes on my lower legs. I also developed a bad knee. The joint pains, like the other symptoms, would remit for extended periods, then return.

All these symptoms could have multiple causes; and some, such as joint pain, back pain, tinnitus, and floaters, could be ascribed to the effects of aging. Others, such as chronic fatigue and chronic diarrhea, might be attributed to a nervous disposition. My local physician took this diagnostic tack. I was not prepared to accept this, and sought help elsewhere.

Since my symptoms often coincided with—or worsened during—my intestinal attacks, I sought out a gastroenterologist. An initial suspicion of celiac disease was ruled out, and the blood work was unrevealing. I was treated for a possible, if undetected, parasite I may have acquired in Nepal; this proved no benefit. When my symptoms later intensified, I went to a university clinic, where another gastroenterologist performed a second colonoscopy in response to a "high reading" which he thought was evidence of systemic lupus or some other autoimmune disorders. I twice saw dermatologists to identify the leg rashes, but was told I had waited too long for a successful biopsy. My situation seemed hopeless at this point.

My worst year was 2008. My symptoms did not remit, as they had in the past, and I developed peripheral neuropathy and moving pains in my arm, shoulder, neck, and back. My middle fingers stiffened. The bad knee worsened, and I experienced twinging in the hips. Muscle weakness was pronounced; the fatigue was debilitating. Late in the year one eye pinkened, my vision blurred, and I developed a cloud of floaters. I live in a remote location in Alaska. [I experienced] pains and weakness with performing the necessary chores of shoveling and hauling snow; joint pain, moving nerve and muscle pains, peripheral neuropathy, and—of course—all those years of chronic fatigue. I remembered the tick rash—a "eureka" moment. A check on the Internet revealed that Lyme disease is endemic on the Oregon coast. I also discovered that my rash met all the diagnostic requirements for a Lyme rash; that allergic reactions to tick bites last days, not weeks; and that the Lyme carrier in Oregon is the western black-legged tick, not the Midwestern deer tick I associated with Lyme. I also discovered that I not only had the core Lyme symptoms, but that they also had developed over the years as Lyme disease commonly progresses. I also learned that all my other symptoms—such as intestinal and eye involvement—were consistent with Lyme.

I saw another, less dismissive, physician and requested testing for Lyme disease. The ELISA screen came back negative, as did the IgG Western blot; the IgM Western blot had one positive band, one band short of an overall positive. My physician, fortunately, was aware from past experience of the inadequacy of the tests for later-stage Lyme. She thought I had a good case and, seeing my distress, took pity and prescribed six weeks of doxycycline. After what was likely a Herxheimer reaction, the response was dramatic; the fatigue lifted the second week, and as treatment continued my pains abetted and my intestinal symptoms resolved. Within six weeks following treatment, however, I had a full relapse. My physician judged it to be probable Lyme disease and told me to hightail it to a Lyme clinic for possible intravenous treatment.

In April 2009, Dr. Burton Waisbren clinically diagnosed neurological Lyme disease with central nervous system involvement. Under his care, I began seven weeks of IV ceftriaxone treatment; in addition, I took erythromycin for the suspected Bartonella henselae infection. In the weeks that followed, my pains subsided and my fatigue lifted. By the end of the third week, my intestinal problems resolved, as did my pains from peripheral neuropathy and conjunctivitis in my eyes. A visit to a Lyme-knowledgeable ophthalmologist confirmed the restoration of 20/20 vision and found no evidence of a continuing Lyme eye disorder. Since I had been diagnosed with mild rosacea many years ago, he speculated that the conjunctivitis might be due to a concurrent episode of ocular rosacea. I am treating it as such.

I continue to take a Lyme-level daily dose of doxycycline, both for possible residual Lyme and for ocular rosacea. The run of erythromycin continues. I have diminishing pain in one arm and occasional episodes of peripheral neuropathy. My understanding is that recovery from the pains and neuropathy of late Lyme often takes months, so I am not discouraged by this. I am steadily getting better and, except for the one arm, steadily improving—the pains are gone. My vision remains restored, my deep fatigue has not returned, my mind is clear, and my intestinal symptoms are gone. I think I may have beaten this thing. I cannot be certain, of course, until after finishing antibiotic therapy. But at this time, I sense I have recovered my life.

Note: After eighteen months of taking doxycycline and erythromycin, his symptoms started to recur. He called me from Alaska and I restarted an oral, multi-antibiotic program for chronic Lyme disease. He has scheduled an appointment for October 20111, and we may need to re-start IV therapy.

Patient 35
First Seen: April 30, 2009

In 1989, I saw a case of amyotrophic lateral sclerosis that followed Lyme disease. I followed this up with a study published in *The Lancet* that showed that the sera from fifty-five cases of ALS showed antibodies to Lyme disease in four instances. I suggested in this article that it might be worthwhile to treat early cases of ALS with ceftriaxone. This suggestion was followed up on by other investigators with some encouraging results, but nothing spectacular.

In the early 2000s, Dr. Rothstein, the present "guru" regarding ALS at Johns Hopkins Medical School, demonstrated that ceftriaxone stimulated an enzyme that, by a feedback mechanism, regulated the glutamate level in the central nervous system. He had found that elevated glutamate levels precipitated the central nervous system changes that occur in amyotrophic lateral sclerosis. (He apparently was unaware that I had suggested ceftriaxone be used to treat ALS in 1989 and that several physicians had tried it with indifferent results.)

Based upon his findings, Dr. Rothstein obtained a multimillion-dollar grant from the government to do a multicenter double-blind study regarding the efficacy of ceftriaxone.

This has led new patients with ALS to request treatments by myself without having to participate in a double-blind protocol. Since I have negative feelings about double-blind studies in patients who might be given something that may help them, I have treated a few cases of ALS with ceftriaxone when they had a bona fide tick exposure.

In the case study to be presented, the patient and her daughter chose empiric treatment only after intense discussion in which they realized they were taking a rational empiric treatment that had not been proven to be effective. In our initial attempts in this direction, there have been failure and a few encouraging results.

This sixty-seven-year-old woman who lived in Missouri suffered a tick bite followed by two weeks of flu-like symptoms and muscle pain in 2003. She stated that she never had felt completely well since that time. In 2006, she began to notice what she thought was arthritis of her spine and "arms." In February 2009, she began to have generalized weakness of her lower extremities and some respiratory distress. A diagnosis of amyotrophic lateral sclerosis was made in a medical center and confirmed elsewhere. Progression seemed rapid, and when seen by me, she was on oxygen and having moderate respiratory distress. Her diagnosis of amyotrophic lateral sclerosis had been confirmed at a large Minnesota-based clinic. She was wheelchair bound.

After prolonged discussion with the patient and her family, the members of the family were split on whether she should go ahead with empiric ceftriaxone. The decision was left up to the patient. She opted to go ahead.

On physical examination on the patient's first visit, she was dyspneic and had weakness of both lower extremities to the point that she was wheelchair bound. She was dependent on nasal oxygen given by nasal catheter at a rate of 2 liters per minute.

With the history, the physical exam, and the laboratory studies, it seemed reasonable to make a diagnosis of amyotrophic lateral sclerosis, chronic Lyme disease, and Hashimoto's thyroiditis. Lyme disease studies showed antibodies to Bartonella and Western blot determinations IgG 41 KD++++, 31 KD, and 39 KD.

After prolonged discussion with the patient, the following course of action was decided upon. A PIC line was inserted in the outpatient department at St. Mary's Hospital; the first dose of ceftriaxone was given under medical supervision shortly thereafter. Arrangements were then made, through the help of her daughter, for the following program to be instituted, as given by home-care companies:

1. Intravenous ceftriaxone (4 grams daily), given first in Iowa and then in Camden, Missouri.
2. Armour thyroid (2 grains twice a day by mouth), Ceftin (500 mg twice a day by mouth), gamma globulin (4 cc intramuscularly weekly) for Epstein-Barr, and Valtrex (1000 mg). Blood was drawn every two weeks to monitor therapy. A six-week course of therapy was given over the next six weeks, under the watchful eye of her daughter and doctors in Iowa and Missouri.

There was no evidence of improvement, but the therapy was well tolerated.

For logistic reasons, the patient was placed in a managed-care nursing home in Missouri. Since there was no evidence of improvement and some evidence of progression, the treatment was stopped six weeks after it was started. Her liver enzymes, which were slightly elevated at the start of therapy, never changed significantly, and the laboratory inventory remained normal.

Several weeks after the therapy was stopped, the patient, while in the nursing home, complained of respiratory distress and died rather suddenly.

Any way one looks at it, this woman did not appear to benefit from the treatment. However, she was given some hope, and her daughter appeared to get some solace by the fact that all possible had been done to help her mother.

Patient 36
Last Seen: July 15, 2009

This is one of the first patients I saw with rather classic Lyme disease after I had discovered a relationship between Lyme disease and amyotrophic lateral sclerosis and became interested in the disease. She presented herself late in 1988, after she was bitten by a tick in the Wisconsin Dells. She developed a fever and generalized rash. These symptoms had continued for eight months when she saw me. I made the diagnosis of Lyme disease and documented the diagnosis with a high titer of anti-Lyme antibodies which, at that time, Dr. Johnson of the University of Minnesota was doing for me. I was just starting to study Lyme disease and treated her for three weeks by ceftriaxone given intravenously at St. Mary's Hospital outpatient department. Dr. Johnson had found that ceftriaxone was the most active antibiotic against Lyme disease. There was an excellent clinical response, and she had improvement in the paresthesia of her hands and diplopia. She continued to work at the post office in spite of difficulty with walking.

In early 1989, a diagnosis of multiple sclerosis was made, and she was given a poor prognosis. She then went to a well-known neurologist, who had been following ever since. There had not been a lot of progression of her ataxia, so she continued to work with great difficulty until recently.

In 2005, while trying to find some improvement, she went to Las Vegas for a diagnosis, where a lumbar puncture was said to be normal. At that time, she started seeing a neurologist in Milwaukee and was given Copaxone. She has been on beta interferon and Copaxone since. In addition, she was given a course of prednisone.

She decided to see me, once again, on July 10, 2009. Since 1988, it has been well established, not only by me but by others, that demyelination occurred due to Lyme disease. My screening tests for Lyme disease were negative, but no IGeneX studies were done because of insurance problems. A complicating feature of her history was that her mother and uncle had multiple sclerosis.

At this point, she certainly has the clinical picture of multiple sclerosis with an abnormal evoked optic potential. Based on my experience regarding Lyme disease causing a multiple sclerosis-like picture, I thought it was reasonable for her to receive a two-month course of intravenous ceftriaxone, Ketek, and Diflucan by mouth. This was to be arranged on an outpatient basis under the aegis of her insurance company. They refused to cooperate. She did not return for follow-up after she got their opinion.

Patient 37
First Seen: July 23, 2009

This fifty-nine-year-old Milwaukee woman was exposed to a heavily populated tick area in North Carolina due to her activities regarding rescuing coatis, which are an endangered species of raccoons found in North Carolina and they are known to be infested with ticks. Her serology against Lyme disease was so positive that IGeneX Laboratory purchased her blood and paid for her to come to California to have her blood drawn so they could use it for controls. Her Lyme disease symptoms of fatigue, muscle aches, joint aches, "brain fog," and memory difficulties started after her visit to North Carolina, where she rescued a sick coati.

In June 2009, multiple sclerosis was suspected because of ataxia and an MRI that showed "white spots" associated with this disease. I saw her first on July 23, 2009. She was referred by her very capable internist, who had made the diagnosis of chronic Lyme disease based on Lyme antibodies and Western blot studies done by a reference laboratory. He had ruled out all other possibilities.

He had given 4 grams of ceftriaxone intravenously through a PIC line. Unfortunately, she suffered a pulmonary embolus and clostridium difficile diarrhea. This was treated with heparin and oral Vancomycin. At this point, her internist referred her to me for management. Her Borrelia antibody was 3.57, Western blot (IGeneX) IgG 41 KD, 58 KD; IgM 41 KD.

I agreed with the diagnosis and started her on ceftriaxone (4 gram daily) through a PIC line which had been left in, Ketek (400 mg twice a day), and Diflucan (200 mg twice a week). (On days that Diflucan was given, the Ketek was skipped because Diflucan raises Ketek levels.) She was ordered to have also by mouth Valtrex for an elevated Epstein-Barr titer, and intramuscular gamma globulin (4 ml twice a week) for a low IgM level which was found.

After a month of this, her insurance company abruptly stopped all payments and then canceled her insurance. They did this in spite of documentation supplied to them and a telephone conference I had with one of their physicians who seemed to understand what happened. To make matters worse, her daughter suddenly died, and the patient stated that she could not afford to pay for any more treatments. Fortunately, her longtime empathetic internist agreed to do what he could to help her.

A summary of her laboratory work showed that her antibodies against Lyme disease were elevated at 3.57, and her Western blots were positive (IgG 28, 30, 31, 34, 45; IgM 41, 60). The other very significant finding was an MRI that showed the white spots we have found in eight other patients with central nervous system Lyme disease. Her anti-Lyme antibodies disappeared after her treatments, as did most of the Western blot bands except for the IgG 41. Here was another patient with MRI findings suggestive of multiple sclerosis (see essay 11).

Patient 38
First Seen: September 10, 2009

This resident of a small town in northern Minnesota had a lifetime of tick exposure as he pursued his hobbies of hunting and fishing. He was a respected and active member of his community until mid-2007, when he started to have slurring of his speech, ataxia, and muscle weakness. These symptoms gradually increased until, when his family presented him, he was wheelchair bound, his speech was almost undecipherable, and he had generalized hyporeflexia. Interestingly, underneath it all, he seemed alert.

He had just returned from a prestigious Minnesota clinic, where he was told there was nothing they could do to help him. As far as the family remembered, they did not offer them any ideas as to what might be wrong with him. Accordingly, the family wanted another opinion.

Based on my previous experiences with demyelinating disease and Lyme disease, I felt that Lyme disease probably was the underlying problem.

An IGeneX study showed Western blot of IgG at 28 KD+, 31 KD++++, 30 KD++, 41 KD+, and 45 KD+. IgM Western blot was 41 KD. Studies for ancillary Lyme infections were, for some reason, not done by IGeneX. He brought along an MRI of his brain which, when I looked at it with the head of radiology at St. Mary's Hospital in Milwaukee, showed marked degenerative changes throughout the brain, consistent with severe neuroborreliosis.

I proposed at a family meeting that a program of intravenous anti-Lyme disease treatment should be instituted. Their reactions were mixed, and they said they would think my suggestion over.

Shortly thereafter, I received a call from a physician at the Minnesota State Board of Health. He told me that after they had received the IGeneX report, that they felt the patient had Lyme disease, and that they would contact the family about the matter.

Shortly after this, I heard from a member of the family that they had talked over my recommendations for treatment with the patient's personal physician. His opinion was that if the prestigious clinic in Minnesota had not recommended treatment, it was not necessary. I never heard from the patient or his family since.

After talking it over again with the radiologist at St. Mary's Hospital, I understood somewhat why the clinic advised no treatment. He said that he had never seen so much brain damage on an MRI and doubted that any treatment would have helped this patient. This patient also had obvious demyelinating findings which were consistent with neuroborreliosis (see essay 11).

Patient 39
First Seen: November 2009

This forty-one-year-old woman presented herself with the following symptoms that started in the fall of 2006: fatigue, joint aches, muscle pain, symptoms of celiac disease, and hair loss. Over a three-year period, her allergist and rheumatologist had been unable to diagnose or help her. She went to the Internet and she self-diagnosed chronic Lyme disease. She lived in a tick-infested area and had numerous tick bites.

I did not repeat her numerous negative studies, but did order an IGeneX Lyme panel. In this panel, she had antibodies against Borrelia. Studies for Ehrlichia, Bartonella, and Babesia were negative. Her physical examination was negative. A Lyme questionnaire that she had found on the Internet was suggestive of Lyme disease. Her IGeneX study regarding the Western blot showed positive blots at IgM 23, 31, and 41 KD, and at 41 KD IgG. Accordingly, I ordered an empiric trial of doxycycline (100 mg by mouth three times a day), erythromycin (500 mg by mouth twice a day), and Diflucan (200 mg by mouth three times a week). (I was not aware of erythromycin and Diflucan interactions at that time.) After a month, there was no response to this program.

Accordingly, I outlined a program that I would try to arrange for her. For a month, she was to take intravenous ceftriaxone (6 grams a day), erythromycin (500 mg three times a day by mouth), and Diflucan (200 mg three times a week by mouth). She was to take 4 cc of gamma globulin intramuscularly weekly.

I never heard from her again, but to my surprise on July 9, 2010, I received the enclosed letter from a nurse practitioner that she had chosen to take over. I felt that changing to rifampicin and Ceftin was reasonable and showed some sophistication of the nurse practitioner. I had told the patient that I did not feel comfortable with having a nurse practitioner who I did not know administer my suggested program, but I admit that according to the letter I received, everything seemed to turn out well. I never heard from the patient after I wrote out the program in January 2010.

The letter from the nurse practitioner was as follows:

I have thoroughly enjoyed working with this patient, while actively participating in the care and treatment of her chronic illness and Lyme disease. Since we have been working together, the patient has regained her cognitive abilities, reduced her migratory myalgias and arthralgias, and has reversed her uveitis. Her energy level has been restored to normal. Tachycardia and insomnia have been resolved. She continues to struggle with neuropathy, primarily in the mornings, which lessens throughout the day. She also continues with cyclic fevers and swollen glands.

The patient has undergone sixteen weeks of IV Rocephin with cyclic oral antibiotics pulsed in during treatment. She is currently on a regimen of rifampicin (300 mg daily) and Ceftin (500 mg twice daily).

She has tested positive for several viral illnesses and has been treated with acyclovir (400 mg twice daily). Naltrexone is assisting in controlling the multiple myalgias and arthralgias. [Apparently, the nurse practitioner had looked at my website regarding naltrexone.]

She takes many different herbal and vitamin supplements. We are beginning to wean her off of some of these therapies in order to assess what is needed at this time. I feel her immune system is functioning properly, and therefore she will need less support. The goal is to have her use supplements which are necessary to sustain her 90% recovery level that she is currently experiencing.

Patient 40
First Seen: November 11, 2009

This twenty-nine-year-old young man presented himself on November 11, 2009. He was kind enough to type out his chronological history that started in October 2002. From 2002 to 2003, he began having chronic fatigue—he was unable to get out of bed or attend university classes. He was treated with psychiatric drugs, to no avail, between 2002 and 2003, when he began to have headaches, eye pain, and visual disturbances. In September 2005, he was diagnosed, on the basis of a low thyroid–stimulating hormone, as having Graves' disease. He received no help from a ninety-day course of methimazole.

In mid-2006, a sleep study was performed, and he was diagnosed with sleep "inertia." He was given stimulants and other psychiatric drugs which, from his standpoint, "messed up his mind." From April 2007 until September 2007, he could not function as a student and had to discontinue his college education because twitching of the muscles in his face and eyes were considered to be the result of a panic attack. Abdominal pain was also present. A CT scan was read as normal, but when I got a copy, it did show the white spots associated with multiple sclerosis (see essay 11). A colonoscopy and endoscopy were normal.

In September 2007, he self-diagnosed Lyme disease from an Internet research and requested a Western blot test. He felt that it was positive. His primary doctor gave him a twenty-one-day course of oral doxycycline, pursuant to "IDSA guidelines." There was no response to his "brain fog" or other debilitating symptoms. He was referred to a rheumatologist, who instituted therapy for fibromyalgia and gave him Flexeril and injections in the back for trigger points.

In March 2008, while hiking in the Sierra Mountains in California, he had a seizure. He was transferred by Med-Flight to Oakland, California, and was told that he had been in shock. Further studies at a Madison hospital in February 2009 failed to reveal the cause of his intermittent episodes of "brain fog" and ataxia. In August 2009, he was given a twenty-one-day course of intravenous ceftriaxone (2 grams per day). His "brain fog" and intermittent headaches and dizziness seemed to improve, but he still felt disabled mentally and physically.

He presented himself to me on November 11, 2009. Based on his history and IGeneX studies of positive Lyme antibodies (1:40 Borrelia) and Western blot studies of IgG 18 KD+++, 23–25 IND, and 39 KD++ and 41 KD, I suggested to him and his father that he receive a higher dose of ceftriaxone intravenously (6 grams per day) plus by-mouth doxycycline, Ketek (40 mg twice a day) (omitting this drug on the days he got Diflucan), and Diflucan (200 mg twice a week). This was started after there was no clinical response to doxycycline, Ketek, and Diflucan given by mouth for a month.

During the first month of the intravenous program, there was a moderate decrease in "brain fog," fatigue, and muscle weakness. Not being satisfied with this, gamma globulin (4 ml intramuscularly) was added to his program. We all felt (his father is a pharmacist) that after this, the pace of improvement accelerated.

We then started to work on his mentation, which he felt had been dulled by the large dosages of amphetamines he had been given for several years as his disease became chronic. We did this by having him take daily the practice tests in the Kaplan book which was published to prepare one for law boards. He felt that this "ploy" did help his mentation problems.

This is the patient's description of his disease—it is not meant to be testimonial, but rather to share with the reader what a documented case of Lyme disease goes through. As of January 2011, he was back in college, successfully working toward a degree, but he still felt that his mentation had been permanently damaged by the analeptics that he had received over the years. His rendition of his case follows; it speaks for itself:

Recent Medical History
Date of Birth: March 15, 1981
Prepared for: Dr. Burton Waisbren, November 2010

Timeline of symptoms/treatment since 2002

Fall 2002
Began having chronic fatigue symptoms and was extremely tired even after 8–10 hours of sleep. Was unable to get out of bed to attend classes at UW or work. Went in to see doctor and was prescribed Prozac for depression.

Continue to have fatigue symptoms and returned to doctor. Several other combinations of psychiatric drugs were tried. None were helpful.

January 2003
Had an acute case of prostatitis for which I was given Cipro.

Mid-2003
Care was transferred to a psychiatrist. Additional iterations of psych drug cocktails were tried; however, there was no improvement with any of them.

Late 2003
Began having headaches, eye pain, and visual disturbances.

September 2005
Diagnosed with mild hyperthyroidism (low TSH) and was given a low dose of methimazole. Instructed to stop taking methimazole after 90 days, although thyroid levels continued to be monitored. Since then, TSH levels have fluctuated between low end of the reference range or remained slightly outside of reference range. It should also be noted that testosterone levels have been low in the reference range.

Mid-2006
Had sleep study performed and was diagnosed with sleep inertia. I was prescribed stimulants in addition to other psychiatric drugs (combinations > 25). Intense muscle pain and fatigue commenced. Primarily the tissue

affected was along the spine in the thoracic and lumbar regions of the back and through the front to the stomach area.

April 2007
Neurological ticks started and muscles in my face and eyes started to twitch. My arms and legs twitched periodically. I was seen in the urgent care, treated and told it was either a panic attack or acid reflux.

July 2007
Had CT scan, colonoscopy and endoscopy performed resulting from severe muscular pain in the abdomen. Nothing was abnormal.

September 2007
Was officially diagnosed with active Lyme infection after researching on my own and requesting a Western blot be performed (see attached results).

I was given 21 days of oral doxycycline pursuant to the current IDSA guidelines and told that I had received "adequate treatment" by medical primary doctor. Symptoms continued and I requested that I be working with a specialist. I was referred to a physician at the University of Wisconsin Hospitals' infectious diseases department. I was told that was the standard treatment and that I would now be treated for pain symptoms through rheumatology and pain management.

October 2007
Had an echocardiogram to determine if I had any heart valve damage. The cardiology department at UW Hospital reported that I had a "slight irregularity" and that the beat would be slightly off. No further treatment was recommended.

November 2007
Started treatment in rheumatology and was diagnosed with fibromyalgia and rheumatoid arthritis.

December 2007
Began pain management treatment and was prescribed Flexeril to relax muscles. Also began receiving trigger-point injections in back.

2008
Continued treatment in pain management and rheumatology. Had a neurological attack in March 2008 while hiking in the Sierra Nevada Mountains in California. Was transferred via Med-Flight to a hospital in Oakland and was told that I was in shock. I was released the next day.

February 2009
Hospitalized in Madison after going to Meriter Hospital for more neurological episodes. Released the next day after no major complications were uncovered. Was deemed unable to work for 30 days and ordered on medical leave.

August 2009
Neurological complications reappeared and I began to lose track of where I was, I would black out, and my legs would sometimes buckle and I'd have problems with stairs and standing up. Twenty-one days of Rocephin treatment (1 gram ceftriaxone) was received daily. Neurological complications started to improve during treatment, but since I ceased treatment in mid-September, feel like they might recur.

October 2009
Shortly after my return from medical leave, I was laid off from my job as a risk management consultant working for credit unions.

November 2009
Began my treatment with Dr. Waisbren after my IGeneX lab panel was extremely positive for Borrelia, Bartonella, and the Epstein-Barr virus. My treatment plan consisted of oral antibiotic medicine including penicillin VK, Valtrex, Ketek, doxycycline, and Diflucan.

February 2010
Commenced intramuscular gamma globulin injections.

March 2010
Began to show signs of physical improvement after several months of treatment. Energy level started to improve after Epstein-Barr virus was treated. Started to train to run 10-kilometer run.

April 2010
Completed 10K "Crazy Legs" run in Madison, Wisconsin. Dr. Waisbren prescribed hydroxychloroquine (antimalarial medicine) for possibility of Babesia treatment.

Summer 2010
Continued antibiotic regimen as prescribed. Physical symptoms showed improvement; however, mental "brain fog" symptoms continued.

September 2010
His PIC line inserted at Columbia St. Mary's Hospital in Milwaukee, Wisconsin. Started 90-day course of ceftriaxone treatment at the rate of 6 grams daily. Continued use of gamma globulin, doxycycline, Ketek, and hydroxychloroquine.

October 2010
Had MRI test performed at UW Hospitals and clinics. MRI findings in all likelihood indicate occurrence of "white plaques" on brain. This is a classic neurological Lyme disease characteristic. Dr. Waisbren will confirm this when the radiologist he works with reviews MRI.

November 2010
Continued signs of improvement mentally. Ability to remember things has improved, and an overall improvement in mood and mental fatigue.

February 2011
I still have not recovered my mentation ability. It was decided to stop all medications since I was still taking ceftriaxone at 6 grams a day, gamma globulin, and doxycycline. The PIC line seemed infected, and we thought this may have been impinging on my recovery; however, all in all, I am better than when we started therapy with IV antibiotics, gamma globulin, and oral antibiotics. Cultures of my PIC line, when it was removed, were negative.

Note: In May 2011, he had gone back into the workforce and was actively working on sales. He feels better than he has "in years."

Patient 41
First Seen: December 10, 2009

This case is of particular interest because, while it does not prove anything, it illustrates a situation in which a patient with established Lyme disease (positive epitope IgG 31 plus Western blot IGeneX of IgM 39 KD and 41 KD; IgG 31 KD, 41 KD, and 51 KD, with a Quest panel being negative), and demyelinating symptoms was apparently cured with just oral therapy.

In addition to his Lyme studies, he has documented antibodies which show that he has some autoimmunity, and he has Raynaud's phenomenon and MRI changes which are consistent with multiple sclerosis, which of course is an autoimmune disease. In addition, he has ataxia, right arm weakness, and absent abdominal reflexes (in my experience, absent abdominal reflexes usually accompany chronic Lyme disease with multiple-sclerosis-type findings). His history is as follows:

This sixty-seven-year-old man was an intrepid deer hunter in northern Wisconsin. He had been chronically ill for three years with fatigue, "brain fog," weakness in his right arm, balance problems, and paresthesias of his feet.

In December 2009, he had noted a rash on his jaw that lasted a month. In June 2009, his physician did a Lyme test which was interpreted as equivocal, and he was given a seven-day course of oral doxycycline. There was no response to this.

On physical examination, a weakness of his right arm was noted. He had ataxia, absent abdominal reflexes, and paresthesias of his feet.

Initial laboratory studies showed a negative Lyme panel by Quest and an elevated antinuclear antibody level. An MRI for multiple sclerosis showed the white spots that we and others have found in multiple sclerosis (see essay 11). In contrast to the Quest studies, IGeneX studies showed IgM Western blot of 39 KD and 41 KD, and IgG studies of 31, 41, and 51 KD. The epitope for IgG 31 was "positive" (IGeneX feels that this is the most revealing test for Lyme disease). In view of the above, he was started on an oral program of doxycycline, clarithromycin, Diflucan, and Valtrex. The Valtrex was used because we have found, almost invariably, high Epstein-Barr titers in chronic Lyme disease, and he did have this finding.

He was started on doxycycline (400 mg per day), clarithromycin (500 mg twice a day), Diflucan (200 mg twice a week), and Valtrex (1000 mg twice a day). Within a month on this program, all of his findings improved, so it was continued. Within another month, he was essentially asymptomatic.

Since then, he has continued on this program, although based upon the renewal records of his antibiotics, I am not sure of his compliance. I think he manipulated his dosage based on his perceived symptoms.

When seen January 17, 2011, he was essentially asymptomatic, was jogging every day, and all previously positive findings for multiple sclerosis were negative. He was gradually tapering his antibiotics, and we decided that he would gradually stop all medications. He feels that he does get symptoms which improve when he restarts or increases the dose of his antibiotics. I am not happy with patients who manage their own dosage in drugs, but over the years have learned that in some cases there is no choice.

At any rate, we have here a patient with documented Lyme disease (epitope 39) who has documented autoimmunity (ANA titer and MRI abnormalities) who, over a two-year period of somewhat sporadic therapy given orally, became almost asymptomatic.

Patient 42
First Seen: December 2009

This thirty-eight-year-old woman was bitten by a tick in December 2007. During the next month, she developed "brain fog," fatigue, generalized joint pain, and muscle pain. She had seen a number of rheumatologists, who were unable to make a definitive diagnosis but had ruled out convincingly lupus and rheumatoid arthritis. Her symptoms became increasingly generalized, and she did not respond to any of the measures ordered by the rheumatologists.

On examination, I was impressed with the organicity of her symptoms in spite of a negative physical examination. Laboratory work showed only a positive Epstein-Barr titer and a Western blot for Lyme disease by Quest of 41 KD. The Quest studies to demonstrate Lyme-related organisms were negative.

I started her empirically on treatment for Lyme disease with oral doxycycline, erythromycin, and Diflucan. She and her husband thought that there was some improvement and that she had had a mild Herxheimer reaction. However, we stopped the program after six weeks when it became apparent to all concerned that we had not significantly helped her symptoms. Of interest was that she had developed a linear rash of a type I had seen with bartonellosis.

On August 15, 2009, we decided to try oral penicillin at 10 grams per day, along with intramuscular gamma globulin (4 ml daily for six weeks), oral doxycycline, and oral Valtrex. There was no clinical response to this, and the patient became increasingly discouraged.

In August 2010, because of the continuance of all her symptoms (i.e., fever, joint pains, fatigue, muscle pain, and "brain fog"), we, with much difficulty, arranged through her insurance carrier for her to have a six-week program of ceftriaxone (6 grams a day intravenously), as well as doxycycline, Ketek, and Diflucan given orally. At the end of three weeks on this program, she, for the first time, was "feeling like herself." We were disappointed when the insurance company cut off their support at the end of four weeks due to a policy they had instituted in regard to the intravenous treatment of Lyme disease. The young couple appealed the decision to stop the treatment, but the program was denied as a result of a consultation with a family-practice physician whom the insurance company selected.

As little as they could afford it, this wonderful young couple decided to "dig into their sock" and pay for the six-week course of therapy I had advised. At that time, the IVs were stopped. She is now being maintained on 10 million units of penicillin VK given daily as she can tolerate it.

When I saw her in follow-up in February 2011, she was asymptomatic and had decided to become pregnant.

Of course, this case does not prove anything, but at least all concerned are satisfied with the results and feel that the attempts were worthwhile. It is disturbing that the national Blue Cross agency that was responsible for her therapy arbitrarily decided on limiting treatment on the advice of a family practice physician, who told me that she had never treated a Lyme disease patient.

Patient 43
First Seen: April 15, 2010

This forty-two-year-old man, who is a nationally known fishing guide, was leading a "Paul Bunyan" life in northern Wisconsin until the summer of 2000, when he sustained a tick bite while deer hunting. This was followed by a circular rash. Since a week after that, he has been chronically ill with fatigue, joint pain, and eventually a case of cardiomyopathy. Two years ago, his constellation of symptoms had reached a point when he was completely disabled and having to lie about at home. Up to that time, he had seen upward of "ten physicians," none of whom were able to make a diagnosis. Included in this group were rheumatologists, gastroenterologists, and internists. Two years before presenting himself to me, he had seen a "Lyme doctor" who made a diagnosis of Lyme disease by a blood test and treated him with a series of antibiotics given sequentially, never more than one at a time. He felt that he may have improved somewhat from the antibiotics, but never enough to leave the house and go back to his beloved profession.

On examination when I saw him on April 15, 2010, he had tenderness over his joints and muscles as well as generalized weakness. Studies showed signs of autoimmunity with elevated ANA titers plus a low gamma globulin. A Quest panel was negative for any Western-blot positives and for Borrelia, Bartonella, Ehrlichia, and Babesia antibodies. His thyroid levels were normal. Clinically, I felt that he had chronic Lyme disease and, as is my practice, started him on doxycycline, Ceftin, erythromycin, and Flagyl.

When I saw him three months later, he had some improvement but still was barely able to leave the house. I added 4 ml of gamma globulin intramuscularly weekly and naltrexone (4.5 mg by mouth twice a day).

When I saw him six months later, his basic metabolic panel was normal and he had improved enough generally to go fishing and to "tune up" for the archery deer season. He and his wife felt that the addition of the gamma globulin and naltrexone had been helpful. I have found in the past that naltrexone (4.5 mg a day) is helpful for the "brain fog" associated with chronic fatigue and Lyme disease.

This is one of the cases that have encouraged me to try oral therapy and gamma globulin before embarking on an intravenous program.

Patient 44
First Seen: April 25, 2010

This fifty-four-year-old woman was bitten by a tick in a part of the country that contained ticks that carry Lyme disease. She developed a bull's-eye rash which she recognized as being consistent with Lyme disease. Two weeks later, she developed chills, intermittent fevers, "brain fog," and a skin rash which was evanescent.

During the next year, she saw a series of physicians who agreed with her diagnosis of Lyme disease. She received intermittent courses of Biaxin, doxycycline, Levaquin, and Ceftin. There were intermittent responses, but in spite of these, she suffered recurrent fevers, "brain fog," joint pains, muscle pains, fatigue, and paresthesias. She had become unable to practice her profession of dentistry. A PIC line had been inserted for a six-week course of vitamin C, but there was no apparent result with this, so the therapy was discontinued.

Tests for Lyme disease, ordered by some of her physicians from IGeneX in California, were said to be "positive."

When seen by me two years after her tick bite, her history was consistent with chronic Lyme disease that had responded somewhat to some antibiotics. However, she had become nonfunctional with fatigue, joint pain, "brain fog," recurrent rashes, and muscle pains.

I felt that she was an emotionally stable woman with bona fide chronic disease which had, during a two-year period, responded intermittently to antibiotic therapy. Her IGeneX studies, done on my initial examination, showed Bartonella 1:20, Babesia negative, Ehrlichia

1:20, IgM and IgG 1:40, Western blot IgG 41 KD, 51 KD, and 31 KD. A plasmid study for B. burgdorferi confirmed by a Western blot was positive. ITF for B. burgdorferi was 1:40. The CD54 was depressed, and she had positive antibodies against the Epstein-Barr virus.

I agreed with the patient that there was enough chance that she had chronic Lyme disease that intense empiric treatment was reasonable. I agreed with her that intermittent attempts had failed to control her Lyme disease. Accordingly, with her agreement, I ordered the following program to be administered in her home state and followed by her personal physician. A PIC line was placed, and she was sent home with the following orders:

1. Daily intravenously 4 grams of ceftriaxone in 50 cc of saline—self-administered after orientation.
2. Doxycycline (100 mg by mouth twice a day).
3. Diflucan (200 mg by mouth twice a week).
4. Ketek (40 mg by mouth twice a day). Skip on days when taking Diflucan.
5. Mepron (700 mg by mouth twice a week).
6. Isoprinosine (500 mg by mouth three times a day).
7. Valtrex (1000 mg daily by mouth).

Her personal physician agreed to oversee the agency selected by her managed-care provider as they instituted the program. All agreed without any red tape. A very good managed-care agency got "on board" and contacted me weekly for four weeks. At that time, the report said that there was some improvement, but that the patient still had fatigue, skin rashes, and paresthesias. The patient had requested that I add sequentially all the modalities I could think of which might help her.

At that time I was starting to add gamma globulin to combat autoimmunity and IV gentamicin and oral Rifampicin to get more bactericidal against Bartonella, to the "mix" of agents that I was using for recalcitrant chronic Lyme disease. Accordingly, I started Gentamicin IV twice a week and Rifampicin 400 mg by mouth daily, and gamma globulin (4 cc intramuscularly) twice a week to the program to be used for this difficult case of chronic Lyme disease. Gentamicin levels were monitored by levels being taken after one of the weekly dosages each week. She and her doctors were warned about ringing in the ears, and because of this, the gentamicin was stopped. The gamma globulin was continued for several months, as far as I can tell. Rifampicin was added for its bactericidal potential against Bartonella.

The patient and the service noted an immediate improvement in fatigue, skin rashes, and muscle and joint pains. The gentamicin was given over a one-month period, but I have no documentation as to how long the gamma globulin was given.

Here we have what might be considered a quintessential antichronic Lyme disease program (i.e., Borrelia—ceftriaxone, doxycycline; Ehrlichia and Bartonella—doxycycline, Ketek). Bartonella is also helped in unreactive cases by giving gentamicin and rifampicin for their bactericidal activity. The low CA57 was treated by the isoprinosine; gamma globulin anti-autoimmunity and potentiating antibiotics; and Babesia by Mepron.

After we stopped the gentamicin, for some reason contact was lost between me, the home-care agency, and the local doctor in charge.

In January 2011, I contacted the patient for follow-up for this book. I was surprised that the intravenous and oral medicines had been at least sporadically continued since the gentamicin was stopped. She and her doctor apparently felt that as long as things were going well, everything should be continued. She added that the PIC line was giving her trouble and would be taken out and that the intravenous ceftriaxone be stopped.

I told the patient that I had thought that the IV had been stopped and that I would appreciate the opportunity to see her again. She consented, and I saw her on February 8, 2011. She said that all symptoms had abated and that she had resumed a normal professional life.

This case, while it fortunately turned out all right, buttresses the importance of communication between out-of-state patients and their cooperating physicians.

I hesitated long and hard about sharing this case in this book, but for better or worse, here it is without any claims as to which of the seven agents she received might have helped her. I do not know how the local doctor decided on continuing treatment and am surprised that the home-care agency continued care for a year without specific orders from the doctor who initiated the program, as I had suggested.

Patient 45
First Seen: July 15, 2010

This forty-six-year-old man had a very traditional life of a northern Wisconsin resident until age thirty-one. He had a good job as a manager of a boat sales company and an outdoor life that included hunting, fishing, and water skiing. When he awoke in the morning, he could see deer playing in his backyard. At age thirty-one, something changed that had progressed to complete disability at age forty-six. During this time, he noticed extreme fatigue, myalgias, joint pain, "brain fog," gastrointestinal distress, episodes of fever, and testicular pain. During all of this time, by sheer determination, he continued his full-time job and many of his outdoor activities. He had consulted many health professionals during this time.

One of these, when he was age forty-four, suspected Lyme disease and sent his blood to a New York laboratory where it was felt that his Western blot studies indicated Lyme disease. Three weeks of oral doxycycline did not improve his symptom complex.

When seen by myself, his complaints included "brain fog," myalgias, fatigue, joint pain, severe headaches, episodes of loss of consciousness, visual disturbances, and testicular pain. He had become completely disabled by these complaints and moved in with his brother. Physical examination was inconclusive.

Studies at IGeneX in California revealed antibodies against Bartonella, and Borrelia antibodies were present in his blood. Western blots for Lyme disease of IgG revealed 41 KDA, and IgM revealed 5 positive bands including 41 KDA.

He had become completely disabled because of his symptoms. I made the decision to institute an "all-out program to combat his presumed chronic Lyme disease."

This included the following: 6 grams of ceftriaxone given intravenously daily for eight weeks; and oral doxycycline, Ketek, Diflucan, and Mepron against Babesia organisms. Gamma globulin was to be given intramuscularly. This program is designed to combat Bartonella, Babesia, Epstein-Barr virus, Borrelia, and life-cycle forms of these organisms. It was started with a PIC line at St. Mary's Hospital in Milwaukee, Wisconsin, on August 26, 2010.

There was a definite clinical response to this program. However, his insurance company refused to pay for more than a month of intravenous therapy. We shifted to an oral program of doxycycline, Ketek, and Diflucan while he is appealing the decision of the carrier to deny him the two more months of intravenous therapy that I think are necessary for his type of syndrome. He is appealing the decision of his insurance company to refuse further intravenous and intramuscular therapy.

He feels that he is better than when we started, but he still has multiple complaints. The consultant hired by the insurance company to deny further treatment admitted to me on the phone that she was a family-practice physician who had only read about this disease. Nevertheless, she ruled that no further therapy should be supported.

I have lost contact with this patient.

Patient 46
First Seen: September 24, 2010

I am including this long case report from this thirty-two-year-old woman whose own description of her disease might be considered a classic. I first saw her in September 2010. First will be presented a case history that she brought in with her:

Here is some of my history: I am a 32-year-old single female Caucasian who works as a receptionist in a dental office. I have lived in Lincoln, Nebraska, all my life. My parents and siblings are all in good health. I was very healthy and active, including running, exercising, camping and many other outdoor activities prior to getting sick. I have gone on hiking trips to Colorado, 10 years and 12 years ago, for two weeks at each visit. I have gone fishing in Canada every year for the past 15 years. I have also been to Honduras and other states in the US for vacations.

I started having problems in November 2007. The only problems I had previous to November were circulation problems, such as random heat patches on my legs, feet, and hands, as well as occasionally a blood vessel would pop and then cause bruising on my hands. The only other problem I had was that I had back pain, and this responded to treatment by a chiropractor. X-rays revealed nothing unusual, but my back continues to bother me.

From November 2007 to July 2008, my symptoms seemed to progress at rapid speed. I had swollen lymph nodes on my underarms, neck and groin; my heart felt like it would skip beats/race and I would get sharp chest pains;

I had my first "episode" in April 2008. Basically what happened was exactly what the definition of a focal seizure is. I have these episodes on a regular basis—somewhere between two and six times per month; my eyes twitched for four months straight starting in May and have been twitching off and on since. In June 2008, I was going to bed and my right arm completely blanched and I had no feeling for three minutes. My arm started tingling and I got feeling back in it, but at the same time had numbness in my face and left thigh. The numbness in my face was light, but didn't go away for several days.

Since that time, I get numb in my feet, hands, legs, arms, and face. It varies how numb it gets, and the numbness migrates around my body. The numbness has continued around my body, and my face has been slightly numb to very numb since February 2008. I started getting joint pains in June 2008. The joints affected are usually wrists, ankles, knees, and hips. Sometimes my ankles hurt to the point that it is difficult to walk. My wrists can hurt to the point where it hurts to write. It varies what joints hurt every day. It can be a mild pain to severe, sharp pains. They have continued to hurt to this point.

Fatigue—I have very low energy. It's sometimes hard to make it through the workday and come home. I rarely do activities (movies, social things, etc.). I sometimes take naps at work over lunch, and I have no energy except to do the necessities in life. If I push myself and stay up late a couple of nights, it takes a few days to "recover." Headaches—I get them frequently.

Other symptoms that I've had for the past 1½ years: I am very forgetful, have terrible short-term memory, severe muscle pains, muscle spasms, altered taste at times, and trouble formulating thoughts. I have to search for the right words when talking. I get dizzy and very spacey. I've gotten rashes on my neck, chest, back, arms, and legs; problems sleeping, night sweats when I wake up very sweaty; emotionally unstable, panics; and very light periods (they seem to be getting progressively lighter). I had some swelling in body (face, legs, arms, etc.), [which] usually only lasts for a day or two; blotchy on legs, hands, and feet.

Since I went from being very healthy and active to having so many problems, I went to several doctors to figure out what is wrong. The tests I've had include CT scans of the brain, two MRIs of the brain, electroencephalograms, Holter monitors, and much blood work. All tests came back negative. I saw a rheumatologist, infectious disease doctor, and a neurologist for exams. No one could find anything wrong, so I started researching what my problems could be and thought all my symptoms pointed to Lyme disease.

I went to see Dr. _____, who is located in South Carolina. He is a Lyme/HIV and infectious disease–certified doctor. I saw him in July 2008. He diagnosed me with advanced Lyme disease. I had a PIC line placed and received IV antibiotics from October 2008 through February 2009. The antibiotics received through IV included the following: meropenem, clindamycin (I was allergic to this), Zithromax, and Levaquin. While taking the IV antibiotics, I also took (orally) Septra DS, metronidazole, Mepron suspension, artemisinin, and Questran. From February 2009 through September 2009, I have taken oral antibiotics including the following: Septra DS, Zithromax, Omnicef, minocycline, rifampicin, and Flagyl. Prescriptions I have taken since July 2008 include Ativan, Lamictal, and Neurontin. The recommended supplements that I've taken include alpha-lipoic acid, coenzyme Q-10, glutamine, multivitamin, N-acetyl L-cysteine, probiotics, magnesium glycinate, and glutathione.

I have followed the recommended treatment for treating the disease most aggressively and have not seen the results that I was expecting. I do not feel that my symptoms/problems have gotten much better or much worse. I still have all the same problems. They continue to come and go, and are sometimes not so bad and other times very bad. Dr. _____ even said at my last appointment that I was having more trouble than I should, and that I have not responded to the treatment as expected. I quit treatment with Dr. _____ in September 2009, mostly because I no longer could tolerate the medications. I started throwing up all of the prescription medications and supplements I took. Also, I wanted to know how effective the Neurontin, Ativan, and Lamictal were. Since I couldn't keep them down anyway, I decided to wean myself off and realized that my problems were not substantially better while taking medications. Since September 2009 I have been off all medication, except Advil and Tylenol for migraines. I went to a hyperbaric oxygen center in January 2010 for four weeks and had hyperbaric oxygen treatment. I did not notice any good effects from this.

I saw Dr. Waisbren, who I found on the Internet, in Milwaukee on September 24, 2010.

On September 24, 2010, after reading over a large volume of medical records brought in by this patient and a case summary that introduced this case report and listening to her long history, I examined the patient. The only positive findings on physical examination, which included a careful neurologic exam, were generalized muscle and joint tenderness as well as scattered lymphadenopathy. I agreed with the diagnosis of chronic Lyme disease. Not wanting to try an intravenous program because the patient lived in Montana and had exhausted the medical help in her community, I suggested that we try an oral program first.

I outlined the program as follows and emphasized that skipping a day or two on a quality-of-life basis would be acceptable. She was to phase in each medication at two-week intervals. She refused further lab studies.

1. Oral penicillin (8 grams per day, spacing in a pill every 8 hours). This was to penetrate the blood-brain barrier and get at the Borrelia.
2. Doxycycline (100 mg by mouth twice a day) for Borrelia and Ehrlichia.
3. Azithromycin (500 mg twice a day) for the bartonellosis.
4. Diflucan (200 mg by mouth twice a week) for cystic phase of Borrelia.
5. Gamma globulin (4 cc twice a week for three months) for autoimmunity.

I called her for follow-up in a month, and she said that she was instituting the program. I then called her on March 17, 2011. She had not kept in touch with me as requested. She said that she had followed the program to the best of her ability and had tapered the intramuscular gamma globulin to every other week. The most important thing she told me was that the focal seizures that had resisted efforts by a series of neurologists had disappeared. Her complaints of fatigue, "brain fog," and muscular/joint pains were no worse and might even have been improved. I decided to add rifampicin (300 mg by mouth) to the mix for its bactericidal effect on Bartonella.

This is a case illustrative of "one size does not fit all in treating Lyme disease" in patients who do not live in close proximity to their physicians.

The case is included because the disappearance of focal seizures seemed worthy of note. This case also illustrates the oral program that is now being phased in due to difficulties in having third parties cooperate in the institution of intravenous therapy.

Patient 47
First Seen: October 7, 2010

On October 18, 2008, while the sixty-year-old patient was in Lyme country in Wisconsin, he suffered a tick bite that was followed by a characteristic rash. He consulted his physician, who sent him for a "Lyme test" at a laboratory next to his office. However, no record has ever been found regarding that lab test. Within ten days after the tick bite, the patient, who had never been seriously ill in the past, developed a stiff neck that was sequentially followed during the next two years with excessive fatigue, short-term memory loss, ataxia, lack of coordination, and night sweats. During the ensuing three years, he has seen a succession of physicians who did numerous tests ($65,000 worth of them), with no diagnosis having been made except chronic depression.

Before seeing me, he had requested a "Lyme test," and this showed antibodies against Borrelia. Western blot tests by this laboratory also were positive, but were interpreted as not being significant because not enough bands were present. He then made an appointment to see me. His history and exposure were so typical that I concurred with him that he had chronic Lyme disease. Initial laboratory tests at Quest showed antibodies against Borrelia, Western blot IgG 46 KD, and an elevated Epstein-Barr. Quest studies for associated diseases were all negative.

We then decided on going to an intravenous ceftriaxone program without trying oral antibiotics, because he had been very intolerant of oral antibiotics in the past. A program that included ceftriaxone (intravenously in a dosage of 6 grams per day), oral Ketek and Diflucan, and intramuscular gamma globulin (4 ml per week) was instituted through an intravenous organization selected by his insurance carrier. The gamma globulin was for the demyelination aspect of his history. An MRI done prior to my seeing him showed the white spots we have seen in other patients in this series (see essay 11). During the first month, he noticed some improvement of his symptom complex of memory loss, fatigue, panic attacks, and joint and muscle pains, so we decided to continue for a total of three months.

However, in January 2011, he developed a generalized reaction to the gamma globulin which necessitated intravenous and oral corticosteroids. We then started a sequential oral program that was to include doxycycline, Ketek, and Diflucan. Within a week, his diarrhea, which had improved while he was on the intravenous program, returned, so everything was stopped. When seen on February 3, 2011, he was functionally disabled because of memory problems, ataxia, and recurrent episodes of dyspnea, sweating, and tachycardia. At that time, we decided to continue the Ketek and Diflucan, which he was tolerating.

Comment: Certainly this case up to now has been disappointing. The next step will be a lumbar puncture regarding demyelination serology and microscopic studies for the search for anatomical evidence of disease. We then will perhaps use empirical treatment for demyelination, as pointed to by the ataxia and his absent abdominal reflexes which we have found in the past to be associated with multiple sclerosis and demyelination.

When seen in May 2011, his brain fog and mentation difficulties had increased to the point that he was unable to function. We decided to restart an IV program using 8 grams of ceftrioxone and supplementing it with IV penicillin G, rifampicin and then IV gentamycin. He is tolerating this IV program well as of September 2011.

Patient 48
First Seen: January 10, 2011

This thirty-six-year-old professor of geology went to Iceland in March 2002 to study their climate. While there, after drinking unpasteurized milk from a famous breed of cows in Iceland, she experienced the following symptoms: bloating, daily diarrhea, vision changes, episodes of paresthesia, and most important, severe fatigue that has interfered with her professional life to this day. The acute symptoms lasted six months. During the ensuing eleven years, the fatigue which she fights daily to keep up a brilliant career has been her main complaint, with the gastrointestinal complaints lurking in the background.

As an academician in a prestigious university, she has seen a succession of physicians during the past eleven years. Lyme disease studied by one expert in the disease lead him to treat her with Minocin, azithromycin, Flagyl, Levaquin, Plaquenil, and Mepron. These have seemed to help some of her symptoms, but she continues to feel unwell and/or have extreme fatigue. Physical examination was unrevealing.

She wanted to postpone further laboratory studies, in view of the many she had over the years. She presented herself because of her Lyme disease, which she was blaming for her overwhelming fatigue. It has gotten to the point that it had infringed on the quality of her life.

The first thing that occurred to me was that antibodies used to diagnose Lyme disease represent reaction to exposure, but not necessarily Lyme disease (see essay 6).

The history that stuck in my mind was that the onset occurred after she drank unpasteurized milk in Iceland. When this was investigated, I found that in Iceland, the sheep and cattle had an endemic disease called Johne's disease which was caused by a paratuberculosis organism. Sheep, but not cattle, are immunized against this disease in Iceland. Paratuberculosis organisms recently have been suggested by some to be a causative organism in Crohn's disease. Cattle interests around the globe have vigorously denied this is the case. Preliminary inquiries about Johne's disease causing human disease have met with vigorous denial, but in this case, it seems reasonable that this possibility be followed up by testing the herd involved and doing paratuberculosis serology tests on the patient. This will be a tedious endeavor because of the fear of the cattle industry that if it is true, it will hurt their business.

A recent study by the Fry laboratory in Arizona was reported as showing both bacteria and bartonella in her blood. She is mulling over whether to undergo further treatment based on this report.

While I try to tool up to investigate this, we decided to empirically treat her overwhelming fatigue with the medications I have found to help some cases of chronic fatigue. These are gamma globulin, Valtrex, and isoprinosine (see www.waisbrenclinic.com).

She has received, in the past, Minocin, azithromycin, Flagyl, Levaquin, Plaquenil, and Mepron. If indeed she has paratuberculosis, the Plaquenil and Mepron might have been of help to her because of her Lyme studies done before I saw her. I felt that when I received the entire laboratory picture of this patient, and considered her travel, empirical treatment for chronic Lyme disease may have been an option. I have communicated this to her but we have lost contact.

Patient 49
First Seen: December 15, 2010

This twenty-nine-year-old cement finisher was in perfect health until, at age twenty-five, he was bitten by a tick while working in Minnesota. He developed a large bull's-eye rash. Several days later, he developed a generalized rash which has continued to the present in spite of numerous treatments suggested by a series of dermatologists. Since that bite, during the past four years, he has had "brain fog," has felt "lousy," and barely can function due to fatigue. Associated with this generalized debilitating illness were joint pain and what he called skeletal weakness. Last year, while vacationing in Hawaii, he met a young physician who suggested that he might have Lyme disease. He frequently had panic attacks. He has recently developed chills and fever. He has continued to "muddle through," but with a new baby on the way, he is determined to get well and back to his normal self.

He searched the Web and became convinced that he had Lyme disease. He saw a "Lyme physician" in his home state of Oregon, who suggested oriental herbs but did nothing more. On the basis of my website, he came to see me. Complete physical examination showed a rash I have come to recognize as probably due to bartonellosis. During a four-hour session, I gave him my course in "Lyme disease 101" and gave him two options:

1. A trial of multiple medicines orally.

2. Three months of empiric treatment with intravenous ceftriaxone, oral doxycycline, Ketek, and Diflucan, along with intramuscular gamma globulin.

Laboratory work via IGeneX showed Borrelia antibody 1:80; IgM Western blot 41, 40; plasmid Borrelia positive; CD57 3.4 (which is low); Babesia negative; and Bartonella 1:80.

In view of the difficulties obtaining a PIC line in Montana, where he is now living, we then opted for an initial oral program which consisted of

1. Penicillin (10 million units by mouth daily) to attack the cell wall of the Borrelia.
2. Doxycycline (100 mg by mouth twice a day).
3. Biaxin (500 mg by mouth twice a day).
4. Diflucan (200 mg by mouth twice a week).
5. Rifampicin (300 mg by mouth twice a day).

He started this program on January 1, 2011. I contacted him in March 2011. He said that he had sequentially instituted the program with a physician in Montana and that he is feeling much better. In view of his subjective improvement, we decided to hold the Mepron (750 mg by mouth twice a week).

Due to the distance involved and less-than-good communication, we decided to continue the oral medications until his wife had their baby at the end of May 2011. He promised to come in for reevaluation after that time. He told me that the monitoring lab work that I suggested was normal. In mid-May, he reported by phone that he was feeling better and that he wanted to continue the oral program. His wife's pregnancy resulted in delivering a healthy baby boy.

One is never comfortable trying to help a patient with whom he is not able to communicate regularly because of long distances. However, this case illustrates the oral approach that is discussed in other parts of this book.

Patient 50
First Seen: November 9, 2010

The patient, age 68, gave this account of her illness:

In May 2006, after returning from a two-week trip in Peru, during which I had slept in the desert and awoke in the morning covered with bites from sand flies. A few weeks later, I noted a deep vertical crease in my forehead which went from my eyebrows to my forehead. Over the next four weeks, these areas began to itch and the skin began to change. During the past four years, I have been to a dermatologist, for whom I used to work [she is a nurse], and he was unable to make a diagnosis of the lesion on my face and neck. In July 2009, I developed 3-cm lymph nodes below my jaw on the left. Biopsy of the skin lesions and lymph nodes revealed necrotizing granulomata which were read as "nonspecific."

Between 2006 and the time she was seen by me in November 2010, she developed severe fatigue which was unusual for her in the past. She continued to have lesions of her face and shoulders.

She searched for a diagnosis at several specialty clinics where, after multiple tests, no diagnosis was made. In 2008, she consulted a "Lyme doctor," who found, at the Fry Laboratory in Scottsdale, Arizona, organisms affixed to red blood cells that were suggestive of Bartonella. IGeneX Western blot studies were positive at 41 KD+++. However, studies at a famous Minnesota clinic were negative for bartonellosis, as were studies for antibodies at Fry Laboratory. In addition, she had borderline-low gamma globulin.

My history revealed, in addition to the Peru trip during which she had multiple fly bites, some difficulty in seeing, increasing muscle and joint pains, and ataxia. Her rash looked to me like that I had seen in "cat scratch fever," and the lymph nodes were consistent with this diagnosis as well.

In view of the fact that she had not responded to a traditional program for Lyme disease, that the study in Scottsdale suggested Bartonella, and that the extensive studies at several specialty clinics had not come up with a diagnosis, I felt that an empiric trial of therapy for Bartonella was a reasonable course to take. Prior to starting this, I suggested that we both look at the Internet regarding the antibiotic sensitivities of Bartonella. To our surprise, we found that in Peru, where she had been bitten by sand flies in 2006, Bartonella was endemic and was caused by sand fly bites. It has been found in many inhabitants of Peru. A search of the literature found that strains of Bartonella from Peru were most sensitive to gentamicin and rifampicin, both bactericidal antibiotics. My studies with gentamicin made me somewhat leery of this drug to start with, so we decided on an empiric trial of antibiotics with better safety records. If they did not cause a clinical response, our plan B was to use intramuscular gentamicin and oral rifampicin. Prior to this, we decided on studies regarding demyelination, because her sight, paresthesias, and ataxia suggested a demyelination aspect. A lumbar puncture showed a low titer for antimyelin antibodies. An optic evoked potential showed optic neuritis, even though at the time the study was done, there were few sight symptoms.

She was started on an antibiotic program that included chloramphenicol, clindamycin, Cipro, and doxycycline. When seen a month later, she felt somewhat better and her chronic skin rash had improved. At that point, I suggested that we consider a course of intravenous therapy that would include gentamicin, rifampicin, and ceftriaxone. She stated that she would talk this over with her Lyme doctor, and I have not heard from her since.

Patient 51
First Seen: November 15, 2010
Age 65

The presentation of this case seemed very characteristic of the chronic Lyme disease syndrome. It may be of special interest because a rapid clinical result followed an oral program outlined in Essay 10. There was a recurrence a month after the initial therapy was stopped. She then responded to a second course of oral therapy after suffering two weeks of a severe Herxheimer reaction. Details are as follows:

In 2000 the patient noted an infected tick bite that was followed by a rash which was diagnosed as Glover's syndrome, a rare skin condition of unknown etiology. A skin biopsy at that time showed the lesion to be infiltrated with T-cells. This was consistent with a diagnosis of Glover's syndrome.

She had the rash intermittently and got used to it until June 25, 2010, when she sustained a tick bite on her upper right arm while living in Madison, Wisconsin. The bite was followed by swelling in the area. She described a bulls-eye rash that appeared.

In mid-July she began to feel "flu-like" and developed a chronic illness consisting of severe fatigue, brain fog, headache, chills and feve4r, and joint and muscle aches. All the symptoms progressed and she became disabled in that she could not continue her active lifestyle.

I saw her in October 2010, and based on her history the following laboratory studies were done:

An IGeneX study on November 15, 2010, showed the following:

1. Western blot IgG 31 KDg, epitope test positive (the lab feels this is diagnostic of Lyme disease)
2. Western blot IgM 41 KD+
3. Western blot IgG 51 KD++, 51 KD+
4. Antibodies to Borrelia by ELISA .12
5. CD57 lymphocytes NK 1.53, which was depressed and is a sign of lack of resistance to Lyme disease

After a thorough orientation discussion we decided to empirically treat presumptive chronic Lyme disease with oral doxycycline, Ketek, Plaquenil, Diflucan, and oral penicillin in the dosages outlined in our oral protocol. She tolerated the oral program well and within a month was asymptomatic and her rash had cleared. She continued the oral antibiotics until mid-February when, against my better judgment, I accepted her decision to stop all therapy to see what would happen.

What happened was that in May, 2011 all of her symptoms returned. However, the rash did not return. I would have been inclined to start an intravenous protocol but she and her husband opted to try an oral program first.

Accordingly, she was started on oral rifampicin, 400 mg BID, oral penicillin of 10 ML units per day, doxycycline 100 mg BID, biaxin 500 mg BID and merpron 400 mg twice a week. Several days after this program was started she developed a Herxheimer reaction that consisted of fever, muscle and joint pains and fatigue. She continued on taking the oral medications and after two weeks the Herxheimer reaction abated and she became asymptomatic. She has continued on the oral program as of September, 2011. A Fry test done at the time of her recurrence was reported as showing high values of Babesia and bartonella.

This case illustrated that one size does not fit all in Lyme disease management and that letting the patient's wishes influence management sometimes ends up to be a satisfactory resolution.

PART TWO

Essays* Regarding Chronic Lyme Disease Syndrome

---

* Essay: An analysis or literary composition dealing with a subject from a limited point of view. (*Merriam Webster's Dictionary*, 10th edition)

Essay 1
A War against Ticks as a Means to Prevent Lyme Disease

In view of the types of experience presented in the case reports in this book, it appears obvious that actions to prevent Lyme disease are in order.

Ticks, the vectors of this disease, must be attacked vigorously. Some of the ways that this can be done are as follows:

When persons, children or grownups, go into a tick-invaded area, whether to play, hike, bicycle, hunt, or fish, they should use a repellent on their clothes that will protect them from ticks. All campsites, whether state, local, or private, should have for sale on the premises tick repellents, along with a brochure outlining how after each exposure, a tick search of the body should be done.

Parents whose backyards are adjacent to "tick areas" should routinely check their children for tick bites each night before they go to bed. People whose backyards are adjacent to "tick areas" should rid the backyards of mice that carry the ticks. Their exterminator should spread cotton balls with anti-mouse poisons in their backyards. The mice use the cotton balls impregnated with mouse poison to build their nests. This simple maneuver will rid the backyard of tick-carrying mice.

Deer hunters often take the deer they have shot to be dressed by butchers who, during the season, pile up the carcasses in their yards. These bodies must be sprayed with tick repellants daily.

Backyards in which ticks reside may be made free of ticks by raising as pets guinea fowl. These fowl will clear the backyards of ticks by eating literally millions of them each day.

In addition, some have suggested that decreasing the population of wild deer might help decrease Lyme disease. I doubt whether this suggestion will be acted upon.

Dogs are notorious carriers of deer ticks. In fact, many veterinarians keep doxycycline on hand to heal Lyme disease in dogs. Accordingly, dogs that live in a house that is in a tick area should have a tick search made every night.

Collectors of wild animals and those who try to save wild animals should be aware that some raccoon species carry ticks. These reside in North Carolina. Before rescued animals are made pets, they should be de-ticked (see patient report 37).

All of the above suggestions above should prevent some cases of Lyme disease.

Another maneuver that might help is the development of a *safe* Lyme vaccine. Problems in this regard will be discussed in essay 2.

Essay 2
Some Words of Warning about the "New" Lyme Disease Vaccine

Having been involved in the study of vaccine complications for years, I cannot resist a few words in this regard.

Between 1980 and 1984 I observed that multiple sclerosis followed in some instances the swine flu vaccine. I also observed that multiple sclerosis and other autoimmune syndromes seemed to follow the Hepatitis B vaccinations. It took until 2004 for it to be published in the *American Journal of Epidemiology* that those who got a hepatitis-B vaccine increased their chance of getting multiple sclerosis threefold.

These observations have been amply confirmed in other literature. The common denominator in acquired autoimmunity following vaccination is apparently a phenomenon called molecular mimicry. Molecular mimicry is defined as "acquired autoimmunity caused by homology between host antigens and antigens introduced by one means or another into the host." An immunologic adjuvant must be present. In this phenomenon when hosts are exposed by the penetration of antigens that contain polypeptides that are present in some organs of their bodies, they mount an autoimmune attack against these organs.

In the case of Lyme disease and presumably its borellia vaccine, the spirochetes inject an antigen capable of causing molecular mimicry. This may explain the autoimmune aspects of chronic Lyme disease (See Essay 11). The potential problems that may be present in a new Lyme disease vaccine is that we know not whether it can cause molecular mimicry and cause autoimmunity and we know not whether it can cause circulating with myelin T-cells which were so brilliantly demonstrated by Dr. Martin and his colleagues at the NIH in Action, MS. (see reference)

One or both of these phenomenons might have caused the autoimmune reactions that forced the withdrawal from the market of the first Lyme disease vaccine. It is my hope that the national Lyme disease "family" will not accept the new Lyme disease vaccine until these two potential charges are faced up to and studied, i.e.: molecular mimicry and evocation of anti-myelin T-cells. In view of this, it seems reasonable to insist that any new Lyme vaccine presented to the public must be devoid of peptides that mimic those present in humans. As far as I know, no consideration of this suggestion has been given by those who seem ready to introduce a new Lyme vaccine.

Essay 3
Testimony regarding Viral Vaccines and Their Dangers, Given by Dr. Burton Waisbren before Congress in 1999*

I would like to thank this committee for the opportunity to share with them my concerns regarding the vaccination policies of the Centers for Disease Control and Prevention (CDC) and the Food and Drug Administration (FDA).

I am a physician and clinical investigator who has practiced internal medicine, infectious disease, and immunology in Milwaukee, Wisconsin, for forty-eight years. No ulterior motives or special interests are responsible for my being here. I am here because I feel an injustice is being done to the children of this country. Included among these children are my sixteen grandchildren.

I want to make it clear from the onset that I fully support hepatitis-B vaccination for individuals who have known risk factors for hepatitis-B infection. The risk factors include sexually active heterosexual adults with more than one sex partner in the prior six months or a history of sexually transmitted disease; homosexual and bisexual men; illicit-injection drug users; persons at occupational risk of infection; hemodialysis patients;

---

*   This essay is included because it illustrates how very long this author has had concerns about vaccines causing autoimmunity disease (By 2011, over one-hundred articles in this regard have appeared.)

household and sex contacts of persons with chronic hepatitis-B infection; and infants born to hepatitis-B-infected women.

My involvement in the field of vaccine toxicity began in 1979 when I discovered that central nervous system demyelination (multiple sclerosis) had been caused, in some individuals, by the swine-flu vaccine. My involvement was heightened when I found the same thing occurred after hepatitis-B vaccination. These findings have been confirmed by many others and have been extended to include other untoward reaction to hepatitis-B vaccine. Reactions include other autoimmune diseases such as rheumatoid arthritis, optic neuritis, post-vaccinal encephalomyelitis, and possibly juvenile diabetes.

An autoimmune disease is defined by the fact that it is caused by the body's immune system turning against its own tissue, be it the central nervous system, the heart, or cartilage. Since the discovery of the autoimmune aspects of the vaccine complications and confirmation of this by numerous investigators, I have been searching the medical literature and studying a number of patients to try to figure out the mechanism or mechanisms by which these autoimmune complications occur. While many explanations have been suggested, the exact mechanism is still unknown. However, this study of the medical literature, of the patients, and of a great number of the reports sent to the *Vaccine Adverse Event Reporting System* (*VAERS*) has convinced me that a serious, perhaps unique problem exists in regard to the toxicity of the hepatitis-B vaccine. There are at least sixteen articles* in the peer-reviewed medical literature about the occurrence of diseases of autoimmunity such as multiple sclerosis after hepatitis-B vaccination. The editors of the renowned medical journals in which these articles appear felt these cases should be brought to the attention of the medical profession. There are thousands, *yes thousands*, of reports by health professionals to the *VAERS* that adverse events have occurred after hepatitis-B vaccination. I am aware of dozens of cases brought against pharmaceutical companies because of damage due to the hepatitis-B vaccine. Many of these cases have been settled with the proviso that the settlements remain a secret.

The fact that these well-established adverse reactions to hepatitis-B vaccine have not been acknowledged or are being denied by both the

CDC and the FDA, is the root cause of the concerns I am about to share with you now.

The first concern is that caused by the experiment sponsored by the CDC which is designed to determine if vaccination at birth of all babies in the United States will eventually decrease the frequency of cancer of the liver caused by hepatitis-B infection. To arrive at the end point of this experiment will take many years.

This experiment is based on the following assumptions:

1. **The vaccine is safe and effective.** While the vaccine is effective, we all know that no vaccine is entirely safe as evidenced by the above-mentioned information.

2. **Five to twenty percent of the people in the United States will eventually contract hepatitis-B infection.** I doubt these statistics.

3. **Up to 25 percent of patients with hepatitis-B infection cannot remember where they got the disease.** Isn't it understandable that the people with the risk factors such as multiple sex partners and injected drug use will not be able to pinpoint where and when they were exposed to the disease?

4. **There is no other way to control hepatitis-B infection in the United States.** Does anyone in this room agree that there is ever only one way to accomplish a purpose?

I hope that this committee will ask for an independent analysis of these rationales.

This brings up my second concern. That is, how can an experiment such as universal hepatitis-B vaccination be adopted nationwide without congressional involvement or approval? Apparently this was accomplished by the joint efforts of an official of an agency that stood to gain much influence and power by the program and by an executive of a drug company which stood to make billions of dollars by the project. What techniques were used and were conflicts of interest involved? Were the rights of parents and children infringed upon?

My third concern lies in the fact that the FDA has apparently not been reacting to the many theories in the medical literature regarding the causes of neurologic complications of vaccination. The FDA does not ask if proposed vaccines exhibit molecular mimicry with human tissue. They do not ask if a vaccine exhibits complementarily with common viruses that may be in the patients. They have not demanded that the HLA patterns of patients who have untoward results be determined. They have not encouraged the development of synthetic vaccines that contain only immunogenic antigens and nothing else. I am concerned that we may see the same or similar adverse reactions to new vaccines. The new Lyme vaccine is a case in point, since that vaccine has more theoretic dangers than does the hepatitis-B vaccine because of the autoimmune nature of the disease itself [in 1999].

When the material I have presented here is considered en toto, I believe it indicates that the present universal hepatitis-B vaccination experiment being conducted in the United States should be abruptly halted for the following reasons:

1. It appears likely that serious untoward events, particularly of the nervous system, have followed the vaccination.
2. In view of this, it is reasonable to suppose that some babies who have little or no chance of getting hepatitis B will suffer unnecessary damage to their nervous system.
3. Information regarding the risk/benefit ratio of this vaccine is not known and therefore cannot be given to parents in an informed consent.
4. There is some doubt as to whether the rights of babies are being violated when they are subjected to an experiment, even with their parents' consent.

France has already stopped their program of universal hepatitis-B vaccination of babies because of reports that surfaced about multiple sclerosis following the vaccination. I hope our country will follow their lead. If we do not, I am afraid public confidence in our vaccination programs will decrease. This would be detrimental to the excellent vaccination programs already in place in the United States.

I would like to thank the committee again for allowing me to share my concerns with them. Documentation of all that I have said here is available in the supplemental material I have given this committee.

Note: All that I said in 1999 is in all probability pertinent to the Lyme vaccine that is about to be presented for use.

Essay 4
The "Emperor's New Clothes Syndrome," Chronic Lyme Disease, and the Infectious Disease Society of America (IDSA)

This essay will start with a repeat of the definition of chronic Lyme disease: Chronic Lyme disease is a syndrome that results when individuals who have been inoculated with multiple microorganisms by infected ticks and who have not responded to an initial course of doxycycline develop extreme fatigue, intermittent fever, joint pain, muscle pain, "brain fog," concentration difficulties, skin rashes, and in many instances symptoms of autoimmune disease to the extent that they impinge upon their quality of life.

When one comes face-to-face with patients of this type in whom other diseases are ruled out, it is obvious that something serious is amiss.

It is a conundrum why a group of respected physicians who are members of the Infectious Disease Society of America have not recognized this and have, instead, written a guideline that essentially denies that the syndrome exists. This guideline has resulted in literally hundreds of patients being unable to be treated for chronic Lyme disease.

Conclusions regarding this conundrum may be:

1. The physicians who wrote and signed the guidelines of the Infectious Disease Society of America may have seen what they

expected to see in the manner of the populace described in Hans Christian Andersen's perceptive fairy tale, "The Emperor's New Clothes."

2. Perhaps the authors of the guidelines had too much respect for authority and decided to sign the guidelines based on the opinion of some of the members of the society without having personal involvement in the treatment of the syndrome.

3. Perhaps they were unduly influenced by the expenses incurred in the many factors concerned in the empirical treatment of chronic Lyme disease.

4. Most probably they were influenced by controlled studies in the medical literature, which were based on deductive conclusions rather than inductive conclusions as described by Francis Bacon in 1622. Have they forgotten the well-accepted statistical dictum, "Absence of proof does not equal proof of absence"?

Deductive conclusions in regard to chronic Lyme disease are suspect because there is no way to prove that a person has chronic Lyme disease. Personal observation (inductive) is what has to be relied upon to conclude that an individual has chronic Lyme disease.

In Hans Christian Andersen's story, a little boy turns the tide by yelling, "But the emperor has no clothes!" At the present time, we must await the time when many will yell out, "These patients are sick!"

This point will have to be proven by inductive observational studies of patients subjected to empirical treatment for chronic Lyme disease. For these inductive studies to reach a level of scientific certainty great enough to indicate empirical multifactorial treatment of chronic Lyme disease, physicians will have to once again believe what their patients tell them. To do this, they will have to remove what Claude Bernard referred to as the "double blind" blinders put on their eyes. (Claude Bernard, in 1865, wrote *An Introduction to the Study of Experimental Medicine* where he describes what makes a scientific theory good and what makes a scientist important, a true discoverer.)

The Internet will provide service in this regard if physicians who treat chronic Lyme disease will present to their colleagues and patients detailed case reports regarding this experience on the Internet as well as in the medical literature. Respected medical journals still reluctantly present case reports. Unfortunately, when they do so, they usually warn about anecdotal evidence. In this respect, isn't it ironic that huge numbers of individuals strongly accept ideas based on anecdotes presented in religious tomes and serious literature?

Phillips, in a brilliant critique of the Infectious Disease Society of America guidelines, has separated out numerous observational studies that suggest the occurrence of chronic Lyme disease as described in this essay. There are over one hundred supporting rebuttals from the peer-reviewed medical literature in his essay!

http://www.ilads.org/lyme_disease/media/lyme_video_phillips.html

Essay 5
Microorganisms Involved in Chronic Lyme Disease and their Antimicrobial Sensitivities

The salivary glands of the ticks that inject organisms into people who get Lyme disease contain a group of microorganisms that live in harmony. They apparently are placed into the salivary glands from their homes in deer and mice in their environment. A brief discussion regarding these organisms and their antimicrobial sensitivity follows.

The bellwether organism is a spirochete named Borrelia burgdorferi, after the government scientist who first described it. It is the spirochete whose ability to cause diseases mimics that of its cousin, Treponema pallidum, which causes syphilis. Like syphilis, Borrelia causes primary, secondary, and tertiary syndromes—first a local rash, when it occurs, which is analogous to a chancre in syphilis. A secondary phase occurs as a rash, which is similar to that seen in secondary syphilis. Then later on, a debilitating central nervous system invasion occurs, which is akin to tertiary syphilis.

This spirochete, as are most spirochetes, is clinically sensitive to the tetracyclines and to the penicillins. Apparently, however, the blood-brain barrier prevents penicillin from entering the central nervous system. This explains why relatively high intravenous doses of penicillins or ceftriaxone are necessary to eradicate Borrelia that resides in the central nervous system. The tetracyclines are not tolerated well enough when given in maximum doses by the oral or intramuscular route to be given by this route for central nervous system Borrelia.

I note that some are trying to use intramuscular Biaxin derivatives to treat chronic Lyme disease. However, in my opinion, the premiere treatment of chronic Lyme disease must include dosages of cell-wall-acting antibiotics such as the penicillins or ceftriaxone given intravenously. However, the intracellular-acting tetracyclines apparently act successfully in the primary local Lyme disease. Thus, doxycycline is effective when this occurs, but it is not effective in preventing tertiary Lyme disease.

A second group of organisms injected by the ticks is in the rickettsial group. They are Ehrlichia and Bartonella. These are small intracellular, gram-negative bacteria. For the most part, they are sensitive to the erythromycins which work on their intracellular metabolism. The Ehrlichia, which are the organisms in the Rocky Mountain spotted fever family, as far as I know, do respond to most antibiotics in the erythromycin and tetracycline families. Their importance is that antibodies against them are good indicators of tick exposure.

The Bartonella organisms, a third group, are a different story. *Some* of these are sensitive only to bactericidal antibiotics. For this reason, when bartonellosis seems to be persisting, it is necessary to turn to rifampicin by mouth or gentamicin by vein. Persistence of bartonellosis can be indicated by linear rashes or by red cell adherence shown by the Fry test.

The fourth known culprit in chronic Lyme disease is the Babesia organisms. They are protozoa which are malaria-type organisms that only can be expected to respond to antimalarial-type drugs such as Mepron. Antibodies against these organisms can be found in the series of cases reported in this book, but they are rare. Regardless, empirical treatment of recalcitrant Lyme disease with Mepron seems reasonable.

Since the majority of patients in this series had antibodies against the Epstein-Barr virus, we have added a drug active against this virus in the treatment of many of our cases of chronic Lyme disease.

Finally, there is evidence that some of the organisms among those we have discussed have life-cycle forms in which they form cysts which are resistant to most antibiotics. This is why we use antifungal drugs like Diflucan for them.

Finally, I and others have observed that gamma globulin potentiates the activity of many antibiotics as well as being useful against acquired autoimmunity. This is the reason it is used for chronic Lyme disease (see essay 6 and its references).

Essay 6
A Suggestion That It Might Be Worthwhile to Add Gamma Globulin to Treatment Protocols for Chronic Lyme Disease

---

There are three reasons why it might be beneficial to add gamma globulin to treatment protocols for chronic Lyme disease. They are:

1. Gamma globulin has been shown to potentiate the antimicrobial action of antibiotics.[1,2,3]
2. Gamma globulin has been shown to be helpful in the management of the Guillain-Barré syndrome, organ transplant rejection syndrome, and thrombocytopenic purpura.[4,5,6] These are all autoimmune syndromes.
3. We know that Lyme disease has autoimmune aspects because of its proven association with multiple sclerosis, which is known to be autoimmune in nature.[7] (Essay 11)

Because of these three reasons, I am suggesting that gamma globulin be empirically tried in recalcitrant cases of Lyme disease in which antibiotic therapy has been found wanting.

Evaluation of these suggestions will be difficult because it will depend on the time-honored suggestions of Francis Bacon who in 1620 stated that careful observation will be the best avenue with which to evaluate scientific studies.[8] This will occur only if clinicians who try gamma globulin in Lyme disease will share their *observations* with colleagues, patients and their families, through the Internet, and through case reports in the medical literature.

However, there are three noninvasive methods by which possible effects of gamma globulin on Lyme disease can be evaluated.[9,10,11] They are:

1. Serial determinations by MRI studies of the glutamate levels in the brains of Lyme disease patients.[9]
2. Serial determinations of the numbers of the autoimmune T- and B-cells circulating in the blood and cerebral spinal fluid of Lyme disease patients in whom gamma globulin has been added to their management program.[10]
3. In vitro determinations by a tube or agar dilution method of the effects of gamma globulin on the antimicrobial activity of antibiotics against Lyme pathogens. These will be difficult because of the fastidiousness in cultures of the organisms involved.[11]

I doubt whether these studies will be done in the near future because of their expense, difficulty, and the fact that there are those who have convinced themselves and others that chronic Lyme disease is not a problem.[12] Because of this, I hope that those who might be interested in this suggestion will not delay in acting on it until all these studies are completed.

References

1. M. Fisher, "Synergism between Gamma Globulin and Chloromycetin in Treatment of Bacterial Infections," *Antibiotics & Chemotherapy* 1 (1952): 315–332.
2. B. A. Waisbren, "The Treatment of Bacterial Infections with Combinations of Antibiotics and (Intramuscular) Gamma Globulin," *Antibiotics & Chemotherapy* 7 (1957): 322–333.
3. B. A. Waisbren, "Pyogenic Osteomyelitis and Arthritis of the Spine Treated with Antibiotics and Gamma Globulin," *Journal of Bone and Joint Surgery* 42 (1957): 414–429.

4. "Gillian Barré Syndrome—Treatment Overview," http://www.webmd.com/brain/tc/guillain-barre-syndrome-treatment-overview.

5. R. E. Schmitt et al., "High Dose Gamma Globulin Therapy in Adults with Idiopathic Thrombocytic Purpora-Clinical Effects," *Annals of Hematology* 48, Issue 1, 1984.

6. "Intravenous Gamma Globulin (IVG) A Novel Approach to Improve Transplant Rates and Outcomes in Highly HLA_ Sensitized Patients," *American Journal of Transplantation* Vol. 6 (2006): P. 459–466.

7. K. Cavert, "Lyme and MS Having the Same Etiology," http://www.canlyme.com/lymemultiplesclerosis.html.

8. F. Bacon, *Novum Organum,* 1620.

9. R. Scrimivasan, Salasulan, et al., "Evidence of Elevated Glutamate in Multiple Sclerosis using Magnetic Resonance Spectroscopy at 3t.," *Brain* 128 (2005): 1016–1025.

10. R. Martin, B. Gran, Y. Zhao, et al., "Molecular Mimicry and Antigen-Specific T-cell Responses in Multiple Sclerosis and Chronic Lyme Disease," *Journal of Autoimmunity*, Vol. 16, Issue 3, May 2001, P. 187–192.

11. B. A. Waisbren, C. Carr, and J. Dunnetto, "The Tube Dilution Method of Determining Bacterial Sensitivity to Antibiotics," *American Journal of Clinical Pathology*, 21 (1951): P. 884–891.

Essay 7
The Treatment of Amyotrophic Lateral Sclerosis with Anti-Lyme Antibiotics

In 1988, a man called and asked me if amyotrophic lateral sclerosis (ALS) could be caused by Lyme disease. He told me that his mother had developed ALS shortly after she had developed a case of Lyme disease. He asked, since his mother was dying of ALS, if it would be reasonable to treat her ALS with antibiotics used in Lyme disease.

Just at that time, Dr. Johnson at the University of Minnesota had found ceftriaxone to be active against Borrelia (the causative agent of Lyme disease).

I replied that it was not an unreasonable idea and that if his doctor, the family, and the patient agreed, I saw no reason why ceftriaxone should not be tried if everything else had failed. Ten days later, the man reported that all had agreed and that his mother had been started on a ten-day course of ceftriaxone at 2 grams per day, given intravenously.

A week later, he called, much excited, and said that his mother had brightened up considerably. Two weeks later, he reported that his mother had suddenly died. (We know now that she might have had a fatal Herxheimer reaction.)

This got me to thinking about the possibility of ALS and Lyme disease being related. I happen to know that a professor of neurology, Dr. Cashman at the University of Wisconsin–Madison Medical School had been saving sera for ALS patients, hoping that eventually they might come in handy.

I called him, and he agreed to test his one hundred ALS sera for Lyme disease, with the serologic tests being developed by his colleague in the University of Wisconsin Medical School microbiology department.

It was found that six of the ALS sera had antibodies positive for Borrelia (B. A. Waisbren, N. Cashman, R. Schell, R. Johnson, "Borrelia Burgdorferi Antibodies in Amyotrophic Lateral Sclerosis," *The Lancet* 8:2 (85544) (1987):332–333.). We published this finding in *Lancet* with the suggestion that it might be worthwhile to try ceftriaxone in some cases of ALS. This suggestion did not go over very well, but the serologic finding was confirmed by Halperin, et al. (archive, *Neurology* 45-5 (1990): P.586–594). They treated nine patients with ALS in 1987, shortly after my paper, with ceftriaxone and felt that perhaps some had responded. Carelli et al., also treated a few patients with ALS with ceftriaxone in 1994 and reported that it was ineffective (article in the *Journal of Neurological Science* 1, 66).

I heard no more about the suggestion that it might be worthwhile to treat ALS with ceftriaxone until 2001. At that time, I was called by a mycologist in California, who told me that he was privy to a study in which ceftriaxone had been found as only one in a large series of things that have been tried and that helped an animal model of ALS. He did not go into detail, but said that his wife had ALS and had responded well to ceftriaxone. He further said that neurologists in the "South" were using it for this reason, but that they did not want to publicize this fact.

His research assistant had found my 1987 paper in *Lancet*. We exchanged e-mails, but communication was broken off. In 2001, I finally found the research assistant who had originally found my paper. He told me that the mycologist had died. As it turned out, the screening program with which the California mycologist was familiar, also involved Dr. Rothstein, a renowned ALS investigator at Johns Hopkins University Medical School. His experimental model was apparently the one used in the screening program and with which the California mycologist was involved.

Using his experimental model, Dr. Rothstein discovered that elevated glutamate levels in the central nervous system was the cause of the lateral nerve damage in ALS. Glutamate became elevated because of the failure of a feedback enzyme system that controlled the glutamate levels in the central nervous system. Ceftriaxone activated this feedback system.

Dr. Rothstein was able to orchestrate a multicenter double-blind study of ceftriaxone in ALS based on his brilliant research. He apparently was unaware of my suggestion in this regard, made in 1987. Because of my interest in ALS, I have been approached to treat some cases of ALS openly with ceftriaxone. This is because there are those who agree with me that double-blind studies should not be done in fatal diseases when there is a reasonable chance that a treatment might help. (I respect the opinion of those who feel otherwise.) The results in the two patients in this series who I was prevailed upon to treat were inconclusive (cases 20 and 35). They indicate, if nothing else, that ceftriaxone is not a "cure-all."

The role of treating demyelinating diseases for Lyme disease is described in essay 11. A more complete reference list regarding amyotrophic lateral sclerosis and multiple sclerosis can be found on the Waisbren Clinic website.

Essay 8
A Consideration of the Laboratory Diagnosis of Chronic Lyme Disease—Comments about the Western Blot Method

An argument could be made that the laboratory diagnosis of Lyme disease "got off on the wrong foot." This is because antibodies to organisms involved in Lyme disease have become the laboratory tool most used to diagnose Lyme disease. For some reason, antibody titers of various sorts have become equated with active disease, whereas they may only indicate exposure to the disease or resistance to it. We all know that evidence of an antibody response does not indicate an active disease. The fastidiousness of the organisms involved has made it impossible to establish Koch's postulates for chronic Lyme disease.

The Western blot studies, which are essentially antibody studies, do seem to be the most positive finding in clinical Lyme disease, but setting an arbitrary level of these antibodies to diagnose a disease that has not been amenable to Koch's postulates seems open to question. By the same token, ignoring antibody results unless they meet arbitrary levels seems suspect. The vast majority of patients in this series showed some Western blot antibody exposure, but many did not meet the arbitrary limits set.

A step in the right direction in this respect is the effort of some microscopists to see offending organisms in the patients' blood smears.

The importance of these observations will depend on the demonstration of just what these organisms are. The obvious initial use of these observations is that a clinician can see if they disappear after treatment (Fry Laboratory).

We all must remember that in our present state of knowledge, the diagnosis of chronic Lyme disease is a clinical one. Many of the patients who are presented in this series have suffered serious "hurts" when they have been told that they could not have Lyme disease because their "Western blots" did not meet arbitrary limits. The majority of the fifty-one reports in this book of consecutive case reports of the chronic Lyme disease syndrome had Western blots positive, but they did not number enough to meet the arbitrary criteria for significance that have been set.

Essay 9
Experimental Studies "Begging" to be done regarding Lyme Disease

There is no attempt in this book to denigrate studies with hypotheses and experiments regarding chronic Lyme disease. However, the emphasis herein has been upon *observations* that might be helpful to people involved with this disease.

Studies "Begging" to Be Done

1. All organisms involved in chronic Lyme disease should be grown in liquid media, and these cultures should be made available to all those who want to study them. This will be difficult because these organisms are all fastidious in nature.

2. The cultures should be studied in vitro by tube dilution or agar dilution methods, with antimicrobials considered for treatment (see reference section for articles by Dr. Waisbren). The antimicrobials should be studied alone and in combination to determine the minimal inhibitory concentrations (MIC) that will inhibit and kill each organism. Since I first reported these methods in 1951, they have become a standard procedure (see reference section for articles by Dr. Waisbren). What I have designated as observational immunology in 1971 should be done via electron microscopy. What should be observed are interactions between body cells and serum and the organisms

involved in Lyme disease, as well as interactions between the Lyme organism and antimicrobials.

3. Autoimmunity due to chronic Lyme disease should be determined by titering concentrations of T and B cells that interact with myelin in patients suspected of having Lyme disease.

4. Animals that should be amenable to study would be ticks (their salivary gland microorganisms) and field mice that are carriers. It would be relatively easy to see what oral medications might decrease the bacterial Lyme-related flora in ticks and carrier field mice when these animals are treated with antimicrobials.

5. The new classes of microorganisms that are now being demonstrated by Dr. Fry of Scottsdale, Arizona (i.e., XMRV and biofilm organisms), should be searched for.

6. Studies of the genetic makeup of Lyme disease sufferers are in order to see if there is a particular genetic makeup that causes increased sensitivity to the organisms.

Essay 10
Two Protocols to Be Considered for the Treatment of Chronic Lyme Disease Syndrome

The difficulties posed by the intransigent stand taken by the third-party payees have led to a consideration of using an oral program rather than long-term intravenous ceftriaxone, which has been used in many of the cases being reported herein. Particularly unsettling is the arbitrary stand taken by the third parties that state that only twenty days of treatment are indicated for chronic Lyme disease.

Whenever possible, we have used intravenous ceftriaxone, but we use many more weeks than four for the treatment protocol. The length of treatment is individually decided upon on the basis of toleration, response, and the length of time the patients have been sick.

The protocol being used for intravenous ceftriaxone (Rocephin) is as follows:

Intravenous ceftriaxone given through a PIC line in a dosage of 6 to 8 grams of ceftriaxone for at least six weeks, longer if the syndrome has entrenched itself for over a year or if the response is coming along slowly. Concomitantly is added by mouth, at two-week intervals depending on toleration, doxycycline (100 mg twice a day); an erythromycin (erythromycin, Ketek, Biaxin, or generic erythromycins); Diflucan (200 mg twice a week) (erythromycin is not given on days that Diflucan is used); Flagyl (500 mg a day); Valtrex (100 mg twice a day); and gamma globulin (4 cc intramuscularly twice a week). When there has not been a satisfactory clinical response after a Herxheimer reaction may have occurred, we treat Babesia with Mepron (750 mg twice a week) and/or another antimalarial (Primaquine or Malarone). For evidence of intransigent bartonellosis (Bell's palsy of the face and gut, and chronic dermatitis), we first add rifampicin and have, on occasion, used intravenous gentamicin.

The second pathway to be considered is as follows: Oral penicillin and Ceftin are used to make up for the Borrelia cell-wall activity of ceftriaxone when it is given intravenously. This is an important aspect of treatment because one has to get around the blood-brain barrier that apparently protects the Borrelia in the central nervous system.

The package inserts of each drug used can be used to determine dosages. Patients are given the package inserts as well.

When the use of intravenous ceftriaxone is impractical for any number of reasons, oral penicillin given in a dose of 10 grams a day, in capsules made up by a compounding pharmacy, and Ceftin in a dosage of 2 to 4 grams a day, depending on toleration, are used. We have found that 6 to 8 grams of ceftriaxone is well tolerated intravenously, in spite of the small dosage being used by many.

In instituting either of these two programs, one has to consider "quality of life issues" and give patients only what they can tolerate. Monitoring of blood counts and basic metabolic panels at regular intervals is in order.

Nexium and yogurt may help oral toleration. Contingency orders for Clostridium difficile and staphylococci studies of diarrhea should be in the patients' possession, which they should use when and if they develop diarrhea. An EpiPen should also be on hand.

Evaluation of treatment remains clinical and patient observation, although decreases in the Western blot and other antibody reactions are thought by some to indicate a clinical response. It may well be, in the future, that if Dr. Fry can find that his observations of organisms in blood smears decrease after treatment, this may be a helpful way of evaluating therapy. Studies of a series of cases of Lyme disease that are in the literature are suspect because of the lack of accepted criteria for diagnosis of this syndrome. These negative studies can be fitted well into the dogma of "lack of proof is not proof of lack" which, in my opinion, has denied many patients with the clinical Lyme disease syndrome empirical treatment.

Essay 11
Further Consideration of Demyelination (Multiple Sclerosis) and the Chronic Lyme Disease Syndrome

---

The fact that sixteen out of the fifty-one cases reported herein showed findings consistent with a demyelinating disease, and that some of these patients did better than would be expected with their demyelination after they were treated for the presumed chronic Lyme disease syndrome, seems worthy of attention (table 1).

I must explain that perhaps I am ultrasensitive to multiple sclerosis, since I had a clinic dedicated to its treatment with immunotherapy for twenty years. During this time, I saw patients with multiple sclerosis almost daily.[1]

The mechanism by which individuals develop acquired demyelinating disease[1] has been well studied.[2] The mechanism has been postulated to occur when a host is exposed to multiple antigens from compatible invading organisms or by vaccine that contains these multiple antigens. Necessary for the phenomenon to occur must be molecular mimicry between some of the antigens and the host's amino acids and chemical complementarity between the antigens of the invading organisms.[1, 2] All that is further necessary is a physiological or added immunologic adjuvant which can be provided by indigenous muramyl peptides.[3,4]

In Lyme disease, there are plenty of complementary antigens, and the main antigens of Borrelia have molecular mimicry with human neurologic tissue.[4]

This syndrome that I postulate is occurring in demyelination with chronic Lyme disease has been named the MAMA syndrome (*m*ultiple *a*ntigenic-*m*ediated *a*utoimmunity).

Whatever the exact mechanism that explains the observation that sixteen of fifty-one cases of the presumed chronic Lyme disease presented here showed demyelinating signs lends credence to the suggestion that multiple sclerosis occurring in Lyme-exposed individuals might merit empiric treatment for the chronic Lyme disease syndrome (see essay 7).

The finding of "white spots" on the MRI of patients with neuroborreliosis is well known. Brian Fallon, who is considered the "father of chronic borreliosis" at Columbia Medical School, states in review of this subject, "MRI scans among patients with neurologic Lyme disease may reveal white-matter lesions of T2-weighted images that are similar to those seen in demyelinating diseases such as multiple sclerosis.[6] Interestingly, the association of Lyme disease with a diagnosis of multiple sclerosis is well known.[7] Interestingly, none of the MRI reports by the neurologist mentioned in this series mention Lyme disease, although a few of the reports of the "white spots" did mention the possibility of multiple sclerosis.

References

1. B. A. Waisbren, *The Hepatitis-B Vaccination Program in the United States—Lessons for the Future,* 1998, ISBN: 0-9719351-0-6.
2. B. A. Waisbren, "Some Serendipitous Results in the Practice of Investigative Internal Medicine," *Wisconsin State Medical Journal,* 1 (1978): 35–40.
3. B. A. Waisbren, *Adventures in the Practice of Investigative Internal Medicine,* (Trafford, 2008), ISBN 978-1-4251-1238-3, chapter 6, pp. 35–40.

4. J. C. Garcia-Monco, J. L. Coleman, and J. L. Benach, "Antibodies to Myelin Basic Protein in Lyme Disease," *Journal of Infectious Disease* 153(3) (1968): 667–668.

5. E. Aberer, C. Brunner, G. Suchanek, et al., "Molecular Mimicry and Lyme Borreliosis: A Shared Antigenic Determinant between Borrelia Burgdorferi and Human Tissue," *Annals of Neurology* 26(6) (1989): 732–737.

6. B. A. Fallon, "Review of Lyme Neuroborreliosis," http://www.canlyme.com/fallonreview/html.

7. J. Badora-Chmielewska et al., "Lyme Borreliosis and Multiple Sclerosis, a Seroepidemic Study," *Annals of Agricultural Environmental Medicine* (2000): 7141–7142.

Table 1
Cases of Presumed Chronic Lyme Disease Syndrome with Demyelination Aspects (Multiple Sclerosis)

Case #	Ataxia	Paresthesia	Hyper-reflexia	Western blot	Absent abdominal reflex	MRI*	Treatment	Copaxone/Beta interferon
1 (p. 3)	+			41, 39 low CD57	+	+	IV	++ evoked potential optic
3 (p. 10)	+ (LP+)	+		41		+	IV	
4 (p. 13)	+ (LP+)				+		Oral	+ Borrelia AB
5 (p. 16)	+		+	41	+			muscle weakness, lower extremities
9 (p. 26)	+	+	+			+	IV	anti-Borrelia antibodies ++
9, 11 (pp. 26, 33)	+	+	+	41		+	IV	anti-Borrelia AB numbness
16 (p.44)	+	+	+	23, 25, 31, 34, 41	+			lost contact
16 (p. 44) 30 (p. 76)	+	+	+	Positive bands Not available		+	IV	muscle weakness, right side + gamma globulin

Case (pp.)				MRI studies		IV	Comments
30, 31 (pp. 76, 78)	+	+			+		
33 (p. 82)	+	+	+				
36 (p. 91)	+	+			+	IV	Copaxone, hyperbaric oxygen, beta interferon
37 (p. 93)	+			41, 58	+	IV	Borrelia antibodies gamma globulin
38 (p. 95)	+	+	+	28, 31, 30, 41, 43	+		
40 (p. 99)				18, 23, 25	+	IV	Borrelia antibodies
41 (p. 105)	+			39, 41, 51	+		right arm weakness IgG 39 epitope
51 (p. 129)	+	+		46	+		gamma globulin Borrelia antibodies

*When one looks up the MRI findings in multiple sclerosis, the type of "white spots" we have considered in this chart are repeatedly mentioned. As I studied the literature, I could find no specific studies regarding their diagnostic importance. Regardless, I feel that it is worthwhile to record the observation that eleven of the sixteen patients with what I thought was chronic Lyme disease with demyelination had "white spots" on their MRI studies. The fact that a number of these patients appear to have less benign courses than in usual multiple sclerosis after treatment for Lyme disease seems worthy of mention, even though it does not prove anything.

Figure 1

Summary of 16 Patients with Possible Chronic Lyme Disease Syndrome Who Were Included in This Report and Who Had Demyelizing Possibilities

Finding	Number of Patients
Ataxia	15
Paresthesias	7
Hyperreflexia	8
More than one Western blot	7
Absent abdominal reflexes*	5
MRI findings of multiple sclerosis	11
Antibodies against Borrelia	6
Abnormal evoked potential	1
Lumbar puncture findings	2

*I may have been remiss in not recording all the patients I found with absent abdominal reflexes and those who had Epstein-Barr titers. Both of these findings stick in my mind as characteristic of chronic Lyme disease based on my observations that started in 1990. There is not enough data available to prove this, but I will be interested in how many of my colleagues notice the same thing.

PART THREE

Additional References upon Which Many of the
Observations and Suggestions in This Book Are Based

Throughout this book, I have "sprinkled" references that may be of interest to those who want to study the chronic Lyme disease syndrome. This list of references that follows contains mostly studies done by myself. These studies have influenced many of the opinions that I have offered in this book.

1. E. Aberer, C. Brunner, G. Suchanek, H. Klade, A. Barbour, G. Stanek, H. Lassmann, "Molecular Mimicry and Lyme Borreliosis: A Shared Antigenic Determinant between Borrelia Burgdorferi and Human Tissue," *Annals of Neurology* 26(6) (December 1989): 732–737.

2. S. Baig, T. Olsson, B. Hojeberg, H. Link, "Cells Secreting Antibodies to Myelin Basic Protein in Cerebrospinal Fluid of Patients with Lyme Neuroborreliosis," *Neurology* 41(4) (April 1991): 581–587.

3. Z. Dai, H. Lackland, S. Stein, Q. Li, R. Radziewicz, S. Williams, L. H. Sigal, "Molecular Mimicry in Lyme Disease: Monoclonal Antibody H9724 to B. Burgdorferi Flagellin Specifically Detects Chaperonin-HSP60," *Biochemistry Biophysics Acta* 1181(1) (24 March 1993): 97–100.

4. R. J. Dattwyler, J. J. Halperin, H. Pass, B. J. Luft, "Ceftriaxone As Effective Therapy in Refractory Lyme Disease," *Journal of Infectious Diseases* 155(6) (June 1987): 1322–1325.

5. J. Desai, M. Sharief, M. Swash, "Riluzole Has No Acute Effect on Motor Unit Parameters in ALS," supplement 1, *Journal of Neurological Science* 160 (October 1998): S69–72.

6. D. Gay, G. Dick, "Spirochaetes, Lyme Disease, and Multiple Sclerosis," *The Lancet* 2(8508) (20 September 1986): 685.

7. R. Lo, D. J. Menzies, H. Archer, T. J. Cohen, "Complete Heart Block due to Lyme Carditis," *Journal of Invasive Cardiology* 15(6) (June 2003): 367–369.

8. R. Martin, B. Gran, Y. Zhao, S. Markovic-Plese, B. Bielekova, A. Marques, et al., "Molecular Mimicry and Antigen-Specific T Cell Responses in Multiple Sclerosis and Chronic CNS Lyme Disease," *Journal of Autoimmunity* Vol 16(3) (May 2001): P. 187–192.

9. A. R. Pachner, "Borrelia Burgdorferi in the Nervous System: The New 'Great Imitator.'" *Annals of the New York Academy of Sciences* 539 (1988): 56–64.

10. B. A. Waisbren, N. Cashman, R. F. Schell, R. Johnson, "Borrelia Burgdorferi Antibodies and Amyotrophic Lateral Sclerosis," *The Lancet.* 2(8554) (8 August1987): 332–333.

11. B. A. Waisbren, "Infection Control in Total Parenteral Nutrition," archive, *Internal Medicine* 130(7) (July 1978): 1175.

12. B. A. Waisbren, C. Carr, and J. Dunnette, "The Tube Dilution Method of Determining Bacterial Sensitivity to Antibiotics," *American Journal of Clinical Pathology* 21 (September 1951): 884–891.

13. B. A. Waisbren, "Treatment with Large Doses of Penicillin in case of Severe Bacteremia due to Proteus," archive, *Internal Medicine* 91 (January 1953): 138–141.

14. B. A. Waisbren, "Antibiotic Treatment of Bacterial Endocarditis due to Enterococcus: Presentation of a Case and In-Vitro Studies That Show a Potentiating Effect of Erythromycin, Chlortetracycline, and Streptomycin on Some Strains of Enterococci," archive, *Internal Medicine* 94 (November 1954): 846–852.

15. B. A. Waisbren, Introduction to the Section on the Clinical Uses of Neomycin, with Exemplary Case Reports, *Neomycin, Its Nature and Practical Application*, S. A. Waksman, ed., (Baltimore: Williams & Wilkins, 1958), 157–165.

16. B. A. Waisbren, "Some Serendipitous Results of the Practice of Investigative Internal Medicine," *Wisconsin Medical Journal* 77(1) (January 1978): S1–S4.

17. B. A. Waisbren, "The Treatment of Bacterial Infections with the Combination of Antibiotics and Gamma Globulin," *Antibiotics & Chemotherapy* 7(6) (June 1957): 322–333.

18. B. A. Waisbren, "The Rabelaisian School of Treating Severe Infection—A Hopeful Paradigm," *Critical Care Medicine* 3(3) (May–June 1975): 118–122.

19. B. A. Waisbren, "Intensive Treatment of Infections with Antibiotics, Intravenous Gamma Globulin, and Aggressive Therapy," *Medical Counterpoint* 2 (January 1970): 23–32.

20. B. A. Waisbren, D. J. Hurley, K. A. Siegesmund, R. M. Guttman, "Morphologic Expression of the Interactions of Human Lymphocytes and Pseudomonas Aeruginosa as Observed by Scanning Electron Microscopy," *Journal of Infectious Diseases* 139(1) (January 1979): 18–25.